Marijuana

AND

Mental Health

Marijuana

AND

Mental Health

Edited by

Michael T. Compton, M.D., M.P.H.

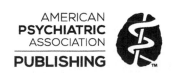

AMERICAN
PSYCHIATRIC
ASSOCIATION
——————
PUBLISHING

If you wish to buy 50 or more copies of the same title, please go to www.appi.org/specialdiscounts for more information.

Copyright © 2016 American Psychiatric Association Publishing

ALL RIGHTS RESERVED

Manufactured in the United States of America on acid-free paper
20   19   18   17   16   5   4   3   2   1
First Edition

Typeset in Adobe's Berkeley and HelveticaNeueLT Std.

American Psychiatric Association Publishing
1000 Wilson Boulevard
Arlington, VA 22209-3901
www.appi.org

Library of Congress Cataloging-in-Publication Data
Names: Compton, Michael T., editor. | American Psychiatric Association, issuing body.
Title: Marijuana and mental health / edited by Michael T. Compton.
Description: First edition. | Arlington, Virginia : American Psychiatric Association Publishing, [2016] | Includes bibliographical references.
Identifiers: LCCN 2015046389 (print) | LCCN 2015047040 (ebook) | ISBN 9781615370085 (pbk. : alk. paper) | ISBN 9781615370658 ()
Subjects: | MESH: Marijuana Smoking | Mental Disorders | Cannabis—drug effects | Cannabinoids | Marijuana Abuse | Psychoses, Substance-Induced
Classification: LCC RC568.C2 (print) | LCC RC568.C2 (ebook) | NLM QV 77.7 |
   DDC 362.29/5—dc23
LC record available at http://lccn.loc.gov/2015046389

British Library Cataloguing in Publication Data
A CIP record is available from the British Library.

Contents

Contributors vii

Preface ix

Acknowledgments xi

1 An Introduction
to Marijuana and Mental Health 1
  Michael T. Compton, M.D., M.P.H.

2 Marijuana's Effects on the Mind
INTOXICATION, EFFECTS ON
COGNITION AND MOTIVATION, AND ADDICTION 11
  David L. Atkinson, M.D.

3 Medical and Recreational Marijuana Policy
FROM PROHIBITION TO THE RISE
OF LEGALIZATION 39
  Arthur Robin Williams, M.D., M.B.E.

4 Medical Marijuana
INDICATIONS, FORMULATIONS,
EFFICACY, AND ADVERSE EFFECTS 71
  Thida Thant, M.D.
  Elin C. Kondrad, M.D.
  Abraham M. Nussbaum, M.D., M.T.S.

5 Marijuana Use and Comorbidity
RISK FOR SUBSTANCE USE DISORDERS AND
ASSOCIATIONS WITH MOOD, ANXIETY, AND
OTHER BEHAVIORAL HEALTH DISORDERS 101

Charles Luther, M.D.
Matthew Lorber, M.D., M.P.A.
Ruth S. Shim, M.D., M.P.H.

6 Marijuana Use and Psychosis
FROM *REEFER MADNESS* TO MARIJUANA USE
AS A COMPONENT CAUSE 119

Claire Ramsay Wan, M.P.H.
Michael T. Compton, M.D., M.P.H.

7 Synthetic Cannabinoids
EMERGENCE, EPIDEMIOLOGY,
CLINICAL EFFECTS, AND MANAGEMENT......... 149

Marc W. Manseau, M.D., M.P.H.

8 Treatment of Marijuana Addiction
CLINICAL ASSESSMENT AND PSYCHOSOCIAL
AND PHARMACOLOGICAL INTERVENTIONS 171

Garrett M. Sparks, M.D., M.S.

9 Prevention of Marijuana Misuse
SCHOOL-, FAMILY-, AND
COMMUNITY-BASED APPROACHES............ 199

W. Alex Mason, Ph.D.
Charles B. Fleming, M.A.
Kevin P. Haggerty, Ph.D., M.S.W.

Index..................................... 227

Contributors

David L. Atkinson, M.D.
Medical Director of Day Treatment Psychiatry, Children's Health; Assistant Professor, Department of Psychiatry, University of Texas–Southwestern, Dallas, Texas

Michael T. Compton, M.D., M.P.H.
Chairman, Department of Psychiatry, Lenox Hill Hospital, New York, New York; Professor, Department of Psychiatry, Hofstra Northwell School of Medicine, Hempstead, New York

Charles B. Fleming, M.A.
Research Scientist, Social Development Research Group, University of Washington, Seattle, Washington

Kevin P. Haggerty, Ph.D., M.S.W.
Director, Social Development Research Group, University of Washington, Seattle, Washington

Elin C. Kondrad, M.D.
Faculty Physician, Saint Joseph Family Medicine Residency, Saint Joseph Hospital, Denver, Colorado

Matthew Lorber, M.D., M.P.A.
Acting Chief, Child and Adolescent Psychiatry, Department of Psychiatry, Lenox Hill Hospital, New York, New York

Charles Luther, M.D.
Assistant Professor of Psychiatry, Department of Psychiatry, Case Western Reserve School of Medicine, Southwest General Health Center Oakview, Middleburg Heights, Ohio

Marc W. Manseau, M.D., M.P.H.
Clinical Assistant Professor, Department of Psychiatry, New York University School of Medicine, and Attending, Outpatient Psychiatry Clinic, Bellevue Hospital Center, New York, New York

W. Alex Mason, Ph.D.
Director of Research, Boys Town National Research Institute for Child and
Family Studies, Boys Town, Nebraska

Abraham M. Nussbaum, M.D., M.T.S.
Director, Adult Inpatient Psychiatry Service, Denver Health Adult Inpatient
Psychiatry; Assistant Professor and Associate Director of Medical Education,
Department of Psychiatry, University of Colorado, Denver, Colorado

Ruth S. Shim, M.D., M.P.H.
Vice Chair, Education and Faculty Development, and Chief of Outpatient
Psychiatric Services, Department of Psychiatry, Lenox Hill Hospital, New
York, New York; Associate Professor, Department of Psychiatry, Hofstra
Northwell School of Medicine, Hempstead, New York

Garrett M. Sparks, M.D., M.S.
Assistant Professor, Department of Psychiatry, University of Pittsburgh
School of Medicine, and Western Psychiatric Institute and Clinic, University
of Pittsburgh Medical Center, Pennsylvania

Thida Thant, M.D.
Resident, PGY-III, Department of Psychiatry, University of Colorado, Au-
rora, Colorado

Claire Ramsay Wan, M.P.H.
Candidate for Master's in Medical Sciences, Physician Assistant Program,
Tufts University School of Medicine, Boston, Massachusetts

Arthur Robin Williams, M.D., M.B.E.
NIDA T32 Fellow, Division on Substance Abuse, Department of Psychiatry, Columbia University, New York State Psychiatric Institute, New York, New York

Disclosures

Elin C. Kondrad, M.D., and Thida Thant, M.D., report that they have no financial relationships to disclose.

Abraham M. Nussbaum, M.D., M.T.S., receives royalties from American Psychiatric Association Publishing and Yale University Press; he has no past or present
financial relationships with marijuana or pharmaceutical industry interests.

Preface

Marijuana affects mental health in diverse ways. Whereas some people would argue that marijuana is beneficial to mental health and well-being, there is very little formal research on this, and *Marijuana and Mental Health* generally sets aside that aspect of marijuana's effects on mental health, instead focusing on the aspects of most relevance to psychiatrists and other health professionals (who rarely see people presumably benefiting from marijuana use but commonly see those experiencing detrimental effects). The goal of all of the contributing authors has been to convey what is known—and specifically what psychiatrists, other mental health professionals, and public health and medical professionals in general need to know—about marijuana and mental health. We do this in just nine chapters. We have been intentionally concise and have striven to be cognizant of the specific information needs of our audience. We have minimized discussions of the storied history of marijuana in America, and we have left in-depth descriptions of physiology, neurobiology, and genetics for other volumes. We also do not discuss the potential health effects of inhalation of smoke itself, which contains numerous carcinogenic compounds (which have been minimally studied in comparison with tobacco smoke). We have chosen to primarily use the word *marijuana* rather than *cannabis*, even if that meant replacing the primary source's terminology of "cannabis" with "marijuana." This was done for consistency and ease of reading and because most laypersons and medical professionals use the word "marijuana."

In one short volume, the authors answer the questions, based on research evidence to date, that health professionals have about marijuana's effects on mental health and mental illnesses. After I provide a brief introduction in Chapter 1, Dr. David L. Atkinson details marijuana's effects with regard to intoxication, neurocognition and motivation, and addiction, in Chapter 2. Given the rapidly evolving policy landscape across the states, Dr. Arthur Robin

Williams covers the current status of decriminalization and legalization of medical and recreational marijuana use in Chapter 3, and Dr. Thida Thant, Dr. Elin C. Kondrad, and Dr. Abraham M. Nussbaum then detail medical marijuana's indications, formulations, efficacy, and adverse effects in Chapter 4. In Chapters 5 and 6, the associations between marijuana and specific mental illnesses are described—Dr. Charles Luther, Dr. Matthew Lorber, and Dr. Ruth S. Shim present the relations between marijuana use and substance use disorders, mood disorders, anxiety disorders, and other behavioral disorders, and Ms. Claire Ramsay Wan and I present the relations between marijuana use and psychotic disorders. Because of the rising threat posed by synthetic cannabinoids, Dr. Marc W. Manseau provides Chapter 7 on the emergence, epidemiology, clinical effects, and management of synthetic cannabinoid use. Chapters 8 and 9 focus on treatment and prevention, respectively; Dr. Garrett M. Sparks gives the latest information on clinical assessment and psychosocial and pharmacological treatments, and Dr. W. Alex Mason, Mr. Charles B. Fleming, and Dr. Kevin P. Haggerty explain school-, family-, and community-based approaches to prevention of marijuana misuse.

It is my hope that our work in compiling the current research on marijuana's effects on mental health will provide clinicians and other interested readers with a thorough but succinct overview of this topic, about which unbiased information is often hard to find. As research in this area advances, the truth will become clearer with regard to the very complex connections between marijuana and mental health.

Michael T. Compton, M.D., M.P.H.

Acknowledgments

Compiling a concise text that conveys the latest clinical knowledge on a controversial topic is a big job, and big jobs are rarely accomplished by an individual woman or man working alone. The compilation of *Marijuana and Mental Health* has been a project whose success is attributable to many. I am especially appreciative of the exceptional staff at American Psychiatric Association Publishing, including John McDuffie, Rebecca Rinehart, Bessie Jones, Robert Hales, M.D., Greg Kuny, Carrie Farnham, Teri-Yaé Yarbrough, and Patrick Hansard. They entrusted me with the heading up of this work and supported me throughout the process. I am particularly indebted to the authors of all of the outstanding chapters, whose individual contributions combine to form a comprehensive, while still clear and concise, text. These authors endured my repeated intrusions into their already very busy professional work, and they honored not only my deadlines but my charge to be wholeheartedly objective and unbiased. Kendrick Hogan endured repeated intrusions into our weekends, accepting this and my other professional passions and always being confident in my ability to orchestrate this book-writing process. I thank Eliana Space for helping me coordinate the tasks of compiling a book written by more than a dozen authors.

The true heroes of this book are the diverse researchers whose work is cited throughout the chapters. Their work, and that of many others, is helping the United States, and indeed the world, to understand the truth about the complex and intricate connections between marijuana use and mental health and mental illnesses. I salute the basic scientists, clinical researchers, addiction treatment specialists, preventionists, public health experts, epidemiologists, and behavioral health services researchers whose work my team of authors and I have summarized here. *Marijuana and Mental Health* serves as a current update of their ongoing work. My hope is that the compilation of their research to date—what is known and what remains to be confirmed or discovered—will reduce ambivalence, equivocation, and controversy and will build consensus that may ultimately help to improve public health and strengthen individuals and communities.

Michael T. Compton, M.D., M.P.H.

CHAPTER 1

An Introduction to Marijuana and Mental Health

Michael T. Compton, M.D., M.P.H.

Clinical Vignette: Anton's Marijuana Use and His Mental Health

Anton Price is a 20-year-old college student who has had a long-standing relationship with a psychiatrist, Dr. Shawn Wrenn. For the past 8 years, Dr. Wrenn has followed Anton—typically seeing him every 3 months, although more frequently during times of slipping academic performance—for mild attention-deficit/hyperactivity disorder and occasional episodes of mild depressive symptoms. Anton is studying philosophy, has connected very well with two of his philosophy professors, and plans to pursue a graduate degree so that he can be a philosophy professor himself. Aside from occasional episodes of mild depressive symptoms that include anhedonia, low motivation, difficulty sleeping, and decreased appetite, Anton is quite social and has many friends. His academic performance has been variable throughout high school and in his first 2 years of college, always passing his courses, although not consistently performing at the level of his parents' and his teachers' and professors' expectations. Dr. Wrenn has prescribed psychostimulants only periodically when Anton's school success has slipped as a result of attentional problems, which primarily affect his test taking; much of their work together has focused on time management, stress management, and strategies for completing homework and taking tests. Although Anton and Dr. Wrenn have always had a therapeutic relationship with apparent openness and good rapport, Anton has only recently told Dr. Wrenn that he consistently smokes "weed for my mental well-being." On hearing this, Dr. Wrenn immediately expressed his concern about the potential effects of marijuana use on Anton's mental health and school performance, but Anton emphasizes that the "Purple Haze weed" that he smokes improves, rather than impairs, his mental health. Specifically, although Dr.

Wrenn points out that smoking marijuana could worsen his amotivation and school performance and lead to addiction and potentially to serious mental health problems, Anton reports that it helps with his appetite and sleep and in making and maintaining close friendships. They both believe that marijuana affects his mental health, but they are not of the same mind regarding how.

A Brief Overview: Plants, Compounds, and the Endocannabinoid System

A Plant Like Few Others

This book is about a plant, although the book says virtually nothing about the plant itself. Instead, the focus is on the effects of ingesting (typically by smoking) the compounds uniquely engineered by the plant and their potential adverse effects on mental health for some who use it. Although the plant itself (*Cannabis sativa*, with subspecies of *sativa* and *indica*) is not a focus of discussion here, it is worth noting that it is one of the most controversial plants in the world; it is highly coveted by many, yet sought out and destroyed by others. It is among a select group of plants, desired by, and having made itself essential to, humans in a way that has guaranteed its survival and proliferation. That is, as articulated by Michael Pollan (2002) in *The Botany of Desire*, this particular plant, now expertly propagated indoors, has hit on an especially ingenious approach to ensuring its survival—by producing chemicals that have the power to alter how humans experience the world.

Marijuana has been illegal in most countries since the 1961 United Nations' Single Convention on Narcotic Drugs (United Nations 1962). According to the U.S. Drug Enforcement Administration (DEA), marijuana is the only major drug of abuse grown within U.S. borders, and the DEA's Domestic Cannabis Eradication/Suppression Program was responsible, in 2014 alone, for the eradication of 3,904,213 cultivated outdoor marijuana plants and 396,620 indoor plants, for a total of 4,300,833 marijuana plants (U.S. Drug Enforcement Administration 2015). This massive effort is met with an equal battalion on the other side of the battle—advocates for the legalization of all plants, and of marijuana in particular.

Delta-9-Tetrahydrocannabinol and Cannabidiol

The marijuana used by many Americans occasionally, or on a weekly, if not daily, basis, comprises more than 400 compounds, including roughly 80 known *cannabinoids,* the chief of which is Δ^9-tetrahydrocannabinol (THC; Borgelt et al. 2013). Given the diversity of cannabinoids found in marijuana, results of studies on marijuana cannot be easily extrapolated to THC itself, and results of research on THC specifically are of only partial relevance to the use of marijuana (D'Souza and Ranganathan 2015). Another key cannabinoid is cannabidiol (CBD), which, unlike THC, does not produce euphoria or intoxication (Martin-Santos et al. 2012).

The various plant strains of *Cannabis sativa* are different, and one joint is different from the next. Furthermore, the cannabinoid composition of the most widely distributed marijuana has varied greatly in recent years and decades and across geographic regions. In the age of engineered cultivation, the THC and CBD content (and the ratio of THC to CBD) of *Cannabis sativa* strains are being fine-tuned, and the resulting products are marketed on the basis of this content and the presumed effects.

The Endocannabinoid System

Researchers have recently begun a long ongoing journey to understand the body's endogenous cannabinoid system and its roles in diverse physical and mental functions. The two main endocannabinoid neuromodulatory lipids are anandamide and 2-arachidonylglycerol, which act on G protein–coupled cannabinoid receptors. Specifically, cannabinoid type 1 (CB_1) receptors are concentrated primarily in the basal ganglia, cerebellum, hippocampus, association cortices, spinal cord, and peripheral nerves, whereas CB_2 receptors are found mainly on cells in the immune system (which may partly explain the effects of cannabinoids on pain and inflammation) (Hill 2015).

In general terms, the endocannabinoid system plays crucial roles in brain development and maturation (e.g., neurogenesis, axon elongation, neural differentiation and migration, glia formation, synaptic pruning), perhaps especially during adolescence and early adulthood (Maccarrone et al. 2014). This underlies the concern about marijuana use in adolescence, which is mentioned in the next section and in subsequent chapters.

CB_1 receptor stimulation has inhibitory effects on neurotransmitter release, and, as such, the endocannabinoid system regulates the release of neurotransmitters. The system plays a role in the regulation of appetite, memory and other domains of cognition, mood, pain, sleep, inflammation, and other physical and mental functions. Whereas the endogenous cannabinoids have very short durations of action, exposure to exogenous cannabinoids (e.g., the THC in smoked marijuana) causes much longer, nonphysiological activation of cannabinoid receptors.

Marijuana in the United States Today

Ambivalence and Controversy

American society is in a state of ambivalence about the beneficial versus detrimental effects of marijuana use. Many Americans view marijuana as a drug like any other drug of abuse, considering it little different from cocaine, the opioids, and other drugs. Many consider it a drug but essentially benign— less addictive and less harmful than alcohol. Another large group of Americans see marijuana as a natural approach to enhancing the senses, improving overall mental health, promoting life satisfaction, deepening connections with spirituality or with friends, treating medical or psychiatric problems, or being helpful in other ways. Opinions about marijuana use are diverse, existing on a broad spectrum (rather than the aforementioned rough categories). Attitudes around the changing landscape of decriminalization (reducing or removing criminal penalties) and legalization (removing criminal penalties and establishing a system of taxation and regulation of production, processing, and distribution)—of both medical marijuana and recreational marijuana—are also varied. Opinions are also changing within individuals and among cohorts; for example, the perceived risk of marijuana use has been decreasing in recent years among youth, which is linked to increasing use rates. There is no current consensus, nor can we expect consensus in the upcoming few years. Just as opinions are changing, in recent decades the marijuana plant itself also has been changing because of selective cultivation and simple genetic modification, resulting in much greater THC levels than the weed of the 1960s peace culture.

Another aspect of the ambivalence in the United States is the glaring nonconsensus with regard to federal law and the evolving laws in states. On the one hand, marijuana is currently classified by the U.S. Food and Drug Administration (FDA) and the DEA as a Schedule I substance on the basis of the Controlled Substances Act, meaning that it has no currently accepted medical use and has a high potential for abuse. On the other hand, many states have passed, and others will pass in upcoming years, legislation allowing for the legalization of medical marijuana programs. These programs allow for the supply and sale of marijuana on the basis of physician recommendation—activities that violate federal law. In fact, in some areas, medical marijuana cards are readily available, there are perhaps more pot shops than coffee shops, and an entire new industry is rapidly evolving. Compounding the lack of consensus, among states that have passed legislation pertaining to some form of legalization, there is remarkable nonconsensus across states in the rules and regulations, or lack thereof, governing medical marijuana programs, driving under the influence, labeling, label accuracy (Vandrey et al. 2015), advertising of edible products, and other aspects of marijuana use.

Health care professionals have had a voice, albeit a limited one, regarding the ongoing ambivalence and controversy. For example, as noted by D'Souza and Ranganathan (2015),

> if the states' initiative to legalize medical marijuana is merely a veiled step toward allowing access to recreational marijuana, then the medical community should be left out of the process, and instead marijuana should be decriminalized. Conversely, if the goal is to make marijuana available for medical purposes, then it is unclear why the approval process should be different from that used for other medications. (p. 2432)

The momentum of pro-marijuana advocacy groups has been remarkable, but there have been few balanced or moderating voices. Meanwhile, federally supported research on marijuana use has focused primarily on detrimental effects while largely ignoring potential health-promoting or therapeutic effects.

Today's ambivalence and controversy are difficult to separate from a long and evolving U.S. history of shifting attitudes toward marijuana. Although not the focus here, the vivid history of marijuana in the United States includes chronicles of both fighting for and fighting marijuana use. In recent decades, the "War on Drugs" centered substantially on marijuana possession and has been heavily critiqued as having been not only a failure of policy but a form of social injustice and oppression. This is detailed by Michelle Alexander (2012) in her thoroughly documented book *The New Jim Crow*, in which she argues that like the era of Jim Crow laws, and slavery before it, the War on Drugs was designed to sustain a racial caste, targeting black men and using the criminal justice system as a contemporary system of racial control. Many people who are advocating for decriminalization (and even legalization) of recreational marijuana use do so on the grounds of the social damage thought to have resulted from the War on Drugs.

Recent Trends in Marijuana Use

Rates of marijuana use are on the rise, as revealed by statistics from a number of epidemiological surveys, including the most recent data from the National Survey on Drug Use and Health (Center for Behavioral Health Statistics and Quality 2015). In 2014, approximately 7.4% of adolescents ages 12–17 were current users of marijuana, equating to about 1.8 million U.S. adolescents. An estimated 19.6% of young adults ages 18–25, or roughly 6.8 million, were current users. Regarding adults age 26 and older, approximately 6.6%

were current users of marijuana, which represents about 13.5 million adults in this age group.

A theme that will be reiterated throughout this book is that the primary concern with regard to marijuana use is that its adverse mental health effects are especially evident among *youth* who use it or when use becomes *heavy*. The available research convincingly shows that individuals who use marijuana regularly—or who begin using it at earlier ages (i.e., adolescence)—are at increased risk for a range of adverse outcomes, including lower educational attainment, unemployment, use of more dangerous illicit drugs, and psychiatric symptoms (Fergusson et al. 2015). At the same time, it must be acknowledged that there exists a substantial proportion of infrequent or even regular (but not heavy) adult users who do not experience harmful consequences as a result of marijuana use.

In addition to concerns about adolescent use and heavy use, using marijuana is also likely to be detrimental among patients with certain psychiatric disorders (e.g., mood, anxiety, psychotic disorders). This is of particular concern for mental health professionals given the high rates of comorbidity between substance use disorders and psychiatric disorders. Although the available research suggests that comorbidity is detrimental, society at large has not yet embraced this conclusion. For example, some states have approved posttraumatic stress disorder (PTSD) as a qualifying condition in their medical marijuana programs, despite the fact that marijuana use appears to be associated with greater, not lesser, PTSD symptom severity; increased risk of violent behavior; and greater alcohol and other substance use among individuals with PTSD (Wilkinson et al. 2015).

What Mental Health Professionals and Other Health Professionals Should Know

Health professionals practicing in states with medical marijuana programs should become familiar with the programs because they undoubtedly will have patients who ask about it. Given that the Controlled Substances Act classification of Schedule I means that, like heroin and lysergic acid diethylamide (LSD), marijuana has no accepted medical use and has a high potential for abuse, physicians cannot legally *prescribe* marijuana. However, in 2013, the U.S. Department of Justice advised U.S. attorneys not to pursue actions against physicians in states that allow medical marijuana. Nonetheless, physicians can only write a letter stating that a patient qualifies for a certification to use the substance, and only after an examination and other requirements.

More high-quality research on marijuana is needed, and to accomplish this, constraints on marijuana research should be reduced, and rigorous research should be funded. Because the ongoing legalization of medical marijuana—and the more recent move toward legalizing recreational marijuana in some states—seems to be minimally informed by science, and because this lack of a scientific basis could in part be due to the difficulty in conducting marijuana research in the United States, federal and state governments have been encouraged to support high-quality research that can then guide policy (D'Souza and Ranganathan 2015).

Research on both medical uses of marijuana-derived compounds and recreational use of marijuana is needed. Reports indicate that there are indeed patients (e.g., those with terminal cancer) for whom marijuana provides relief for symptoms (e.g., nausea and vomiting or pain) that no medication has been able to relieve. It is likely that compounds within marijuana are useful for a number of human health conditions, but research has yet to identify the exact chemical compositions that are most effective or their precise mechanisms of action. Rigorous research is also needed on the effects of recreational use, especially among adolescents. The federal government (specifically the National Institute on Drug Abuse and other institutes within the National Institutes of Health) will be funding a more than $300 million longitudinal brain-imaging study of the effects of marijuana and other drugs on adolescent brain development. This study, the Adolescent Brain Cognitive Development (ABCD) study, will follow approximately 10,000 children beginning at ages 9–10, before initiation of drug use, through the period of highest risk for substance use and other mental health disorders (National Institutes of Health 2015). The ABCD study and other large studies will undoubtedly shed light on the mechanisms by which addictive substances exert both pleasurable effects and detrimental effects on brain development. As noted previously, most people who use marijuana do not develop addiction, but for those who do, addiction is a serious consequence. More research is also needed on factors that predispose individuals to or protect them from addiction in the context of initial or escalating drug exposure or intake.

Things will be changing in the years ahead. Health professionals should expect changes to laws pertaining to driving under the influence, changes to drug-free workplace policies, and major expansions of and changes to medical marijuana programs. Health professionals should also stay tuned for an evolving story pertaining to potential therapeutic uses of CBD. At the time of this writing, 23 states and the District of Columbia have passed laws legalizing medical marijuana, and some 15 additional states have enacted laws allowing access to CBD oil or high-CBD strains of marijuana. Regarding ongoing and upcoming biomedical studies (both preclinical research and clinical trials), CBD is being examined in relation to epilepsy, cancer, pain, spasticity, inflammatory diseases, and diverse behavioral disorders, including anxiety disorders, schizophrenia, and substance use disorders.

Key Points

- The *Cannabis sativa* plant is grown both within and outside of the United States. Marijuana contains roughly 80 known cannabinoids, the chief of which are Δ^9-tetrahydrocannabinol and cannabidiol. They interact with CB_1 receptors in the brain, which are also the targets of endocannabinoids, including anandamide and 2-arachidonylglycerol.
- American society is in a state of ambivalence about the beneficial versus detrimental effects of marijuana use. This ambivalence is apparent in varied and changing opinions and perceptions, the lack of consensus with regard to federal versus state law, and variations among state laws.
- Marijuana use is on the rise, and there is reason for concern with regard to marijuana use among youth or when use becomes heavy. Individuals who use marijuana regularly or who begin using it earlier (i.e., in adolescence) are at increased risk for lower educational attainment, unemployment, use of more dangerous illicit drugs, and psychiatric symptoms.
- Mental health professionals and other health professionals should be aware of medical marijuana programs in their respective states, as well as evolving research and policy pertaining to marijuana.

References

Alexander M: The New Jim Crow: Mass Incarceration in the Age of Colorblindness, Revised Edition. New York, New Press, 2012

Borgelt LM, Franson KL, Nussbaum AM, et al: The pharmacologic and clinical effects of medical cannabis. Pharmacotherapy 33(2):195–209, 2013 23386598

Center for Behavioral Health Statistics and Quality: Behavioral Health Trends in the United States: Results From the 2014 National Survey on Drug Use and Health (HHS Publ No SMA 15-4927, NSDUH Series H-50). Rockville, MD, Substance Abuse and Mental Health Services Administration, 2015

D'Souza DC, Ranganathan M: Medical marijuana: is the cart before the horse? JAMA 313(24):2431–2432, 2015 26103026

Fergusson DM, Boden JM, Horwood LJ: Psychosocial sequelae of cannabis use and implications for policy: findings from the Christchurch Health and Development Study. Soc Psychiatry Psychiatr Epidemiol 50(9):1317–1326, 2015 26006253

Hill KP: Medical marijuana for treatment of chronic pain and other medical and psychiatric problems: a clinical review. JAMA 313(24):2474–2483, 2015 26103031

Maccarrone M, Guzmán M, Mackie K, et al: Programming of neural cells by (endo)cannabinoids: from physiological rules to emerging therapies. Nat Rev Neurosci 15(12):786–801, 2014 25409697

Martin-Santos R, Crippa JA, Batalla A, et al: Acute effects of a single, oral dose of d9-tetrahydrocannabinol (THC) and cannabidiol (CBD) administration in healthy volunteers. Curr Pharm Des 18(32):4966–4979, 2012 22716148

National Institutes of Health: NIH launches landmark study on substance use and adolescent brain development, September 25, 2015. Available at: http://www.nih.gov/news/health/sep2015/nida-25.htm. Accessed November 24, 2015.

Pollan M: The Botany of Desire: A Plant's-Eye View of the World. New York, Random House, 2002

United Nations: Single Convention on Narcotic Drugs, 1961. New York, United Nations, 1962

U.S. Drug Enforcement Administration: Domestic Cannabis Eradication/Suppression Program. Washington, DC, U.S. Drug Enforcement Administration, 2015. Available at: http://www.dea.gov/ops/cannabis.shtml. Accessed Novemer 24, 2015.

Vandrey R, Raber JC, Raber ME, et al: Cannabinoid dose and label accuracy in edible medical cannabis products. JAMA 313(24):2491–2493, 2015 26103034

Wilkinson ST, Stefanovics E, Rosenheck RA: Marijuana use is associated with worse outcomes in symptom severity and violent behavior in patients with posttraumatic stress disorder. J Clin Psychiatry 76(9):1174–1180, 2015

CHAPTER 2

Marijuana's Effects on the Mind

Intoxication, Effects on Cognition and Motivation, and Addiction

David L. Atkinson, M.D.

Marijuana is one of the most commonly abused substances in the world, and it is the most commonly abused illicit substance among youth and adults in the United States and Europe. The human brain is the most sophisticated object in the natural world, and of all animal organs, it requires the most time and most precise orchestration to develop. The effects of Δ^9-tetrahydrocannabinol (THC) on the developing brain can critically alter this developmental process. Regardless of the developmental stage, marijuana can disrupt some of our most valued human faculties—the abilities to test reality, reason, control our impulses, set priorities, relate to others, and reach our goals. How marijuana affects these capacities will be reviewed in this chapter.

Clinical Vignette: Harriet Begins Marijuana Use at Age 13

Dr. Chiara Cervello is a child and adolescent psychiatrist and junior faculty member at an academic medical center. She is evaluating a 14-year-old female patient named Harriet Dolcefoglia, who was admitted to the inpatient unit for suicidal ideation and possible psychosis. Harriet has no psychiatric history apart from evidence of undiagnosed attention-deficit/hyperactivity disorder (ADHD) and increasingly prominent risk-taking behavior developing through early adolescence. Her family history is notable for both parents having used marijuana frequently. Harriet's mother no longer uses, but her father progressed to opioid use and has not been with the family for 6 years because of intimate partner violence directed toward Harriet's mother. Harriet's birth and developmental history are notable only for her mother having used marijuana during pregnancy to "treat nausea…every once in a while." Harriet's mother regrets her choice to use marijuana but does not want to tell her daughter not to use because it would seem hypocritical. Furthermore, a number of media headlines that she has read in the past few years seem to indicate that scientists have proven that marijuana is safe for developing adolescents.

Harriet had no major behavioral problems through grade school, but she had difficulty keeping friends, aside from one or two less popular girls, possibly because of her tendency to playfully annoy her peers. Harriet is intelligent but disorganized in time management and school projects. She learned to anticipate defeat in all of her endeavors, and she occasionally wonders if it would be better not to be alive. She moves around frequently during sleep, often bites her nails and picks scabs on her skin, and either seems disinterested in class or impulsively answers the teacher without raising her hand. Harriet also has frequent headaches and has a variable appetite from day to day, although there are no reported body image issues regarding weight. She went through puberty early, and an older boy took interest in her just before her thirteenth birthday. Her mother allowed her to date because she thought it would improve Harriet's self-esteem. Harriet began to use marijuana with her boyfriend at 13 and progressed to daily use during open-lunch periods in high school at age 14. Harriet's new group of friends in her freshman year of high school consists almost entirely of students who use marijuana.

When Harriet was admitted to the inpatient unit, she was initially diagnosed with bipolar I disorder, single manic episode, severe with psychotic features, because of her rambling, tangential speech with paranoid themes. On the unit, Harriet was irritable, intrusive, and verbally aggressive. She did not sleep during her first night on the inpatient unit. A family history taken by Dr. Cervello shows that Harriet has no family history of bipolar disorder. She also does not display hypersexuality, grandiosity, or decreased need for sleep. Harriet endorses having racing thoughts and occasional paranoia, as well as sleep disturbance and irritability that seemed to have increased during the first 3 days of the hospitalization. After a urine drug screen tested positive for THC, a substance use assessment was done through automated menus in the electronic medical record. Harriet states that she smoked "once or twice a couple of weeks ago" and "didn't remember exactly." During the next 3 days, the irritability, lability, and tangential speech gradually lessen and her psychosis clears.

Harriet's discharge diagnoses are cannabis-induced psychotic disorder and cannabis use disorder, and a substance-specific follow-up handout is given to her mother, who subsequently phones two programs; however, the first is not a working number, and the second program no longer treats adolescents. Harriet is discharged from the hospital on risperidone and is sched-uled for non-substance-specific therapy. She resumes smoking marijuana daily at school, and her emotional lability and irritability toward her mother return, while her grades continue to fall. Harriet's mother threatens to send Harriet to "boot camp" if she does not improve, so Harriet decides to stop using marijuana. Rather than throw the drug away, she decides to "save it for an emergency." Harriet puts an ounce of it in a shoe box, which she then wraps several times with duct tape to prevent herself from opening it impul-sively, and hides the box in her attic.

Shortly thereafter, Harriet's boyfriend starts to date another girl, and one day Harriet arrives home from school distraught about this. She goes up to the attic to retrieve some of the marijuana, and her mother notices this and finds her stash. Her mother notifies Harriet's outpatient counselor, who states that Harriet is in distress and does not want to take away her only "cop-ing skill." Her mother, frustrated by the response, calls Dr. Cervello for help.

Harriet's presentation and psychosocial situation raise a number of ques-tions both for her mother and for Dr. Cervello. Is marijuana truly addictive? Is it "physically addictive?" What is the effect of marijuana on cognitive functioning? What is marijuana's effect on motivation? What role does the age at exposure have in the individual's risk for addiction? What risk does the adolescent user have of transitioning to other substances of abuse? What effects does marijuana exposure have during different developmental stages?

This case touches on the number and diversity of clinical problems an adolescent who uses marijuana might face and present with in the clinical setting. Often, a mental health professional, such as the child and adolescent psychiatrist, is in an uncomfortable position of trying to treat the disorder without sufficient tools at his or her disposal. Other clinicians believe that marijuana is an antidepressant or mood stabilizer, even encouraging their patients to smoke "in moderation." By the very definition of the term, using an *addictive* substance in moderation is difficult. Furthermore, there are some indications that simply moderating use does not greatly reduce depen-dence risk (Swift et al. 2009). Parents concerned about their child's use often receive mixed messages from different clinicians, and very few providers are trained in adolescent substance use.

Acute Intoxication Effects

Marijuana's reinforcing effects are known to involve the same mesolimbic do-pamine system that underlies the reinforcing properties of other substances of abuse (Volkow et al. 2014a). The concept that marijuana is distinct from other illicit drugs is not supported by science; there are well-demonstrated overlaps of the marijuana neural system with the neural systems of other drugs of abuse. THC activates cannabinoid type 1 (CB_1) receptors that are found in multiple brain regions. The shell of the nucleus accumbens and the ventral tegmental area (VTA) are rich in CB_1 receptors (Cooper and Haney 2008). In these areas CB_1 receptors lie on GABAergic inhibitory neurons, very similar to μ opioid receptors. Both CB_1 activation and μ opioid receptor activation inhibit the inhibitory GABA interneurons (Spano et al. 2010) and thus "cut the brake cable" on dopamine release, leading to the same rapid burst firing of dopamine cells that is common to all drugs of abuse. Whereas a steady tonic firing of the dopamine circuit is associated with balance and contentment, the phasic or burst firing of dopamine is associated with subjective "liking" of the drug and the experience of euphoria. Although euphoria is one of the main and most well known properties of using marijuana, it is certainly not the only effect of the drug.

Marijuana's acute intoxication is associated with subjective quickening of associations and euphoria. Higher doses lead to relaxation, decreased motor activity, and a significant sense of calm. As users observe their world, they report perceiving an intense influx of sensory information from ordinary stimuli and are highly focused on internal sensations of the body. Sensory gating is diminished, and the individual may have to avoid strongly stimulating experiences, including bright lights (Iversen 2008).

A coming-down phase occurs after the high, and individuals may describe cravings for food and the sensation of an empty stomach. Rather than craving any type of food, there seems to be a specific craving for the sweet and salty varieties, which is borne out even in animal models. The social aspects of friendship may be enhanced by the chemical euphoria, or the individual may remain contented while socially withdrawn (Iversen 2008).

The euphoric effects can enhance the perception of current activities and can decrease the boredom associated with unexciting tasks. Activation of the mesolimbic dopamine system causes an increase in the *salience* of stimuli, meaning that small things that would not be otherwise important suddenly grab the brain's attention. This may cause the user to focus more on one particular thing, even though executive functioning may be impaired, and hinder appropriate shifting of focus. Also consistent with involvement of the reward pathway, users may develop fantasies of power, including the belief that they have arrived at a transcendent insight (Iversen 2008).

Acute intoxication may also bring about transient sensory experiences and synesthesias (Iversen 2008). There are reports of quicker associations and greater creativity. However, a study testing the hypothesis did not show that moderate-potency marijuana enhanced creativity, measured as divergent thinking, and revealed a decrease in creativity in those who were smoking high-potency marijuana (Kowal et al. 2015).

Marijuana's Effects on IQ, Neurocognition (Including Executive Functioning), and Other Psychological Functions

The links between marijuana use and cognitive deficits generate controversy, but longitudinal studies have shown a reduction in IQ (Meier et al. 2012). This is notable because IQ is generally stable throughout the life span, and any reduction is typically unexpected. The deficits in IQ were actually not shown to be related to socioeconomic factors (Moffitt et al. 2013), as has often been stated. Marijuana's effects on neurocognitive functioning include deficits in processing speed and attention or working memory (Thames et al. 2014), which did not differ between current and past users. Short-term memory tasks are impaired consistently in animal models, and human effects can be substantial, particularly when there is a long period over which the information must be retained and the task becomes increasingly complicated (Iversen 2008). Marijuana use in adolescence and adulthood is associated with effects on other executive functions, sustained attention, and impulse control (Fontes et al. 2011) and also impairments in decision making (Grant et al. 2012). Decision-making dysfunction measured in certain tasks may be related not solely to cognitive processes but also to affective processes. Young marijuana users show not only inefficient information processing but also a tendency to pursue large rewards in their decision making (Solowij et al. 2012). It is very difficult to disentangle the effects of marijuana use from the effects of preexisting temperaments more often seen in marijuana users. However, efforts have been made to minimize this confound, and a large imaging study, the Adolescent Brain Cognitive Development (ABCD) study, has been planned to track youth prior to the onset of marijuana use and through adolescence in order to better understand causality in these associations.

Some individuals report increased focus on one particular task, but this increase in focus is often achieved in a manner disconnected from a more global awareness. They have difficulty tracking conversations over time, particularly as the information becomes more complicated (Iversen 2008). Marijuana has effects on cognition, euphoric or motivational centers, fear circuits, memory, motor circuits, and reality testing. The perception of time may be altered, and there is a tendency for users to do things very slowly and to estimate time intervals poorly (McDonald et al. 2003). Some may experience hallucinations, illusions, or other aspects of impaired reality testing.

Marijuana's Effects on Motivation

One of the greatest areas of interest with regard to the cognitive effects of marijuana is the question of whether marijuana use decreases motivation. The term *amotivational syndrome* has been used colloquially and in the media, but the term has not been regularly used—or the construct adequately studied—in research settings. There is growing evidence that motivation is adversely affected by marijuana use. In an animal model, injection of a CB_1 agonist into the anterior cingulate of rats made them less likely to invest physical effort to obtain a high reward and created a preference for smaller immediate rewards, whereas vehicle injections did not (Khani et al. 2015).

In the short term, decreased locomotor activity, and even states of catalepsy, are evident following THC administration in both humans and animals (Iversen 2008). Users of marijuana often call the experience "couchlock" and believe the phenomenon to be more or less common with different strains of marijuana. The experience of decreased activity may reflect actions on the motor system and may not involve motivation per se. The use of marijuana over time has been associated with general malaise (Brook et al. 2008). As mentioned earlier in this chapter, sleep is a well-documented part of the *coming-down* phase of marijuana (Iversen 2008). The effects of sleep disturbance from cessation of marijuana use are also well established (Bolla et al. 2010), but it is not known to what extent sleep disruption or excessive sleepiness mediates marijuana's effects on energy and motivation.

Decreased motivation may be mediated by marijuana's decreasing of dopaminergic transmission in the striatum (Albrecht et al. 2013; Volkow et al. 2014b). The effects of chronic marijuana use on reactivity to dopamine were studied in a recent positron emission tomography study (Volkow et al. 2014b), which showed decreased reactivity to challenge with methylphenidate (a dopamine reuptake inhibitor). One would expect all drugs of abuse to impair motivation because of their common effects on dopamine (Volkow et al. 2004), and this again raises the question as to whether marijuana is particularly harmful to motivation compared with other substances of abuse. However, direct comparisons suggest marijuana's particular role in decreasing motivation. Data from the Monitoring the Future study indicated that marijuana users reported lower energy and motivation relative to alcohol users, as well as lower school or job performance (Palamar et al. 2014). More research is needed to clarify the exact nature of marijuana's effects on motivation, with particular attention to adolescents, for whom motivation is especially crucial to successful psychosocial development.

Marijuana and Addiction

Intimately connected to the question of motivation is the question of addiction, which itself is a disease of disordered and monopolized motivation. The existence of marijuana addiction has remained a controversial subject in the media. Scientifically, the question has been settled (Budney et al. 2007), and the inclusion of cannabis use disorder in DSM-5 (American Psychiatric Association 2013) is a reflection of established scientific consensus. The fundamental similarities in mechanism of action and addictive phenomena across various substances of abuse suggest the possibility for cross-addiction, gateway effects, and long-term consequences of early exposure.

Marijuana addiction has the same basic process as other addictive disorders (Volkow et al. 2014a). To illustrate the effects on the user, the model of Volkow et al. (2010) is useful to explain the different brain areas involved. The neurobiology of addiction comprises four separate domains: reward salience (nucleus accumbens, ventral pallidum, and medial orbitofrontal cortex), motivation (involving outputs from the accumbens to the motor cortex, cingulate gyrus, dorsal striatum, and orbitofrontal cortex), implicit and contextual memory (amygdala and hippocampus), and control (involving the anterior cingulate and prefrontal cortex).

The initial intoxication has conscious and subconscious effects on the user through the phasic release of dopamine from VTA neurons (Figure 2–1). The dopamine release subconsciously stamps in the experience as pleasurable in the amygdala, and these positive associations are very slow to fade—just as animals remember for a long time where food was located in the past. The bursting euphoria is experienced through the activation of phasic burst firing in the nucleus accumbens shell. This activity colors all marijuana-associated experiences positively with enhanced valuation. Because dopamine signals importance, and not just pleasure, the individual will be more likely to ascribe importance to experiences under the influence of marijuana.

The individual's next encounter with marijuana will lead to subconscious cues being processed as positive, and amygdala inputs will activate the nucleus accumbens core, impelling the person to seek the drug (Figure 2–2). The individual may have conscious memories of the experience, but regardless of conscious valuation, there will be a subconsciously generated tendency to approach the drug while craving is experienced. The nucleus accumbens core will directly activate motor circuits, including the dorsal striatum and motor cortex, and the orbitofrontal cortex will assess the need to

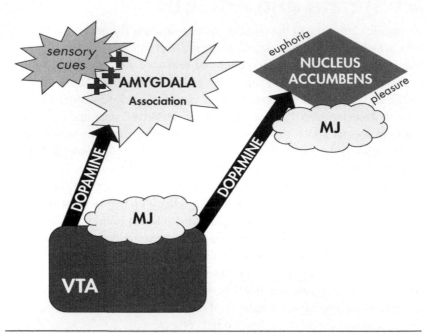

FIGURE 2–1.   Initial intoxication.

Δ^9-tetrahydrocannabinol (THC) causes phasic, burst firing of dopamine by disinhibiting neurons in the nucleus accumbens shell and ventral tegmental area (VTA), simultaneously giving a subjective experience of euphoria (nucleus accumbens shell) and stamping-in positive associations (in the amygdala) of marijuana (MJ) related sensory cues, which become an implicit/subconscious memory (i.e., a *conditioned stimulus*).

go and get the drug. This process is set in motion prior to inhibitory circuits having a chance to act.

In the clinical vignette, each step Harriet takes toward cutting open the shoe box containing her stash is accompanied by anticipatory dopamine firing, pleasurable but not satisfying—priming further craving. Harriet may have a relapse cued by memory of the boyfriend she fears she is losing because he may have become intimately linked in her amygdala as a drug cue. Alternatively, she may crave an enhancement of mood secondary to loneliness and rejection—states marked by disruptions of tonic firing of dopamine. Her craving to use again takes hold strongly before more reflective appraisals are possible. Her negative emotional state might further prime her to stress-induced relapse, partly as a result of the prefrontal cortex not functioning as well under stress.

As Harriet perceives a strong desire to use but also faces the danger of being sent to "boot camp," the anterior cingulate fires on detecting danger or

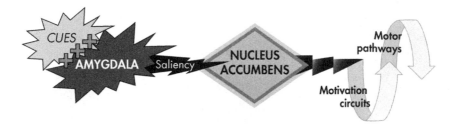

FIGURE 2–2. Drug seeking.
Repeated exposure of marijuana-related cues leads to implicit recognition of a positively conditioned stimulus by the amygdala, resulting in activation of the nucleus accumbens core to subconsciously and automatically initiate the search for the reinforcing drug. The nucleus accumbens core is a limbic-motivational-motor interface and activates drug-seeking behaviors.

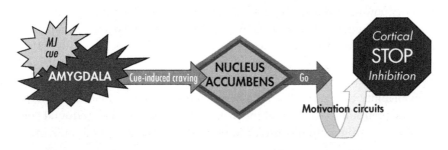

FIGURE 2–3. Inhibition of craving.
The executive control circuits must be activated to inhibit craving from translating into action. This requires active resistance to the urge, involving the inferior frontal cortex, prefrontal cortex, and anterior cingulate cortex.

conflict, and the prefrontal cortex is called into action (Figure 2–3). Finally, the inferior frontal cortex may be able to inhibit the drug seeking that has been activated by the recognition of an approach cue, but the inhibition may not engage in time to thwart the growing desire to seek the drug. Reward and motivation increase with approach to the drug, and the expected reward may overwhelm the brain's inhibitory capacity as steps are taken toward repeated drug use (Figure 2–4). The brain's inhibitory systems may not be able to stop the approach behavior when a reward is more proximate and the reward expectancy is of larger magnitude.

The mesolimbic system of adolescents is highly responsive to reward, and this heightened reward response stands in contrast to the decreased in-

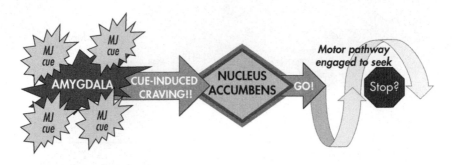

FIGURE 2–4.   Failed inhibition of craving and relapse to drug seeking.
Continuous cue exposure fatigues executive cortical control circuits, while craving
strengthens them; escape from cue-induced craving must occur quickly before reward expectancy increases and cortical control circuits become overwhelmed. A delayed inhibition may not occur in time.

hibitory powers of the incompletely developed prefrontal cortex, placing adolescents at higher risk of impulsive decision making and of choosing highly
rewarding stimuli over safer alternatives (Casey and Jones 2010). Resisting
minor cravings triggered by momentary cues requires willpower, reflected
by activation of the prefrontal cortex. If exposure to drug cues in the context
of availability continues, it will be very difficult for the individual to maintain the prefrontal inhibition of the drug seeking because the prefrontal cortex tends to fatigue from constant inhibition of craving, and the individual
may succumb to use.

Harriet's craving for the drug will grow with repeated use. Addiction involves decreased reward sensitivity coupled with increased reward expectancy
(Volkow et al. 2010). For many users, the drug-related high is perpetually
remembered as the intensely pleasurable high felt during the first experience, termed *euphoric recall,* which leads to the well-known phenomenon of
"chasing the high." This involves attempts to replicate the original high that
has become increasingly impossible to obtain because of desensitization of
dopamine receptors and other compensatory adaptations following excessive activation of the mesolimbic dopamine system. Interestingly, the draw
of the expected reward grows more powerful even as the subjective experience of pleasure gradually diminishes. Individuals may be conscious of taking larger amounts of marijuana, but they often increase use slowly and
subconsciously as the reward becomes less satisfying. Each use raises the reward thresholds and decreases the ability of natural reinforcers to motivate
and appropriately reinforce the individual. Thus, the social praise and sense
of self-efficacy gained from a delayed reinforcer (e.g., getting good grades in

school) evaporate in comparison with the immediate reward received from marijuana use—particularly in the moment of craving.

Repeated drug use causes unnaturally large phasic burst firing of dopamine in this circuit, leading to decreased tonic dopamine firing and downregulation of the system seen in marijuana users (Volkow et al. 2014b). Likewise, the negative emotional states of being hungry, angry, lonely, tired, stressed, and bored are all associated with decreased tonic firing of dopamine and might lead to drug use in an attempt to fill the voids. Unfortunately, repeated intoxication leads to additional episodes of burst firing of dopamine that further destabilize the brain's reward circuitry, and the steady, tonic firing of a contented brain becomes more elusive.

Cannabis Use Disorders: Prevalence and Risks

Addiction to marijuana, termed *cannabis use disorder* in DSM-5, has a past-year prevalence of 3.4% among 12- to 17-year-olds and 4.4% among 18- to 29-year-olds and an estimated lifetime prevalence of 11.8% among men and 5.4% among women in the general population (Khan et al. 2013). Many people believe that the drug has very low addictive potential because the number of individuals who develop cannabis use disorder after having used marijuana at least once is much lower than for other drugs (1:11), although this may be the result of social, legal, and commercial factors and may not be an intrinsic measure of addictive liability. Dose, route of administration, and frequency of use all affect the addictive potential of a substance. It has been suggested that 25%–50% of daily users are dependent (Hall 2015), and among those who did not have cannabis dependence at age 18, those who continue to use heavily beyond age 18 go on to develop addiction (DSM-IV cannabis dependence; American Psychiatric Association 1994) a little over one-third of the time (Swift et al. 2008).

Adolescence is a critical time of brain development during which the individual is learning self-regulation, gathering useful experiences, acquiring knowledge for future productivity, and taking on adultlike social roles. Throughout this learning process, the adolescent is undergoing biological brain changes, particularly in the late-developing prefrontal cortex. A central feature of addiction is that the magnitude of the expected reward grows over time and begins to overcome the brain's control circuits. This imbalance may develop more rapidly in adolescents because they are highly reward responsive and have poorly developed prefrontal circuitry (Casey and Jones 2010). Consequently, adolescent marijuana use is particularly worrisome; one in six adolescent users develop dependence by age 24 (Swift et al. 2008).

In half of the cases of cannabis dependence, the dependence develops within 5 years of first use (Lopez-Quintero et al. 2011), which is shorter than the median 10-year time course for the development of alcohol dependence (Behrendt et al. 2009). Most who develop cannabis dependence do so before they are 25 years old. This may be due to the age at initiation of marijuana use being earlier than for most drugs, with the modal age at initiation of use being only 15 years. Because of the finding that few individuals develop problematic use of marijuana when starting later, some clinicians have encouraged youth to "delay" marijuana use until they are 21 or 25. However, we do not yet have evidence that this strategy is effective in delaying use, much less achieving the end goal of decreased rates of addiction. Twin studies may cast doubt on the utility of this approach. In twins discordant for marijuana use (i.e., when one twin uses marijuana and the other does not), it seems that a marijuana-using co-twin is at higher risk for all substance use disorders. However, when one twin simply uses earlier than the other, the early-using twin is at higher risk of substance experimentation than the late-using co-twin but not of developing DSM-IV cannabis dependence or other substance use disorders (Grant et al. 2010).

Because of these discrepant findings, researchers have debated whether the developing adolescent brain is especially susceptible to addiction following drug exposure, termed the *adolescent vulnerability hypothesis*. Alternatively, the correlation of adolescent exposure and subsequent addiction could be due to a tendency for individuals with higher heritable risk to use substances earlier than those with lower risk, termed *recruitment effects* because those most susceptible to use are "recruited" earlier in life. Genetically informed studies generally suggest that the bulk of the increased risk of addiction seen in adolescent users is due to recruitment effects (Degenhardt et al. 2013). These findings do not rule out the adolescent vulnerability hypothesis, which has been supported in some human studies showing that adolescent marijuana exposure leads to greater risks for dependence on drugs other than marijuana, whereas later exposure does not (Agrawal et al. 2004; Lynskey et al. 2003); adolescent vulnerability to addiction is well demonstrated in animal models (Hurd et al. 2014). Furthermore, there are strong concerns that adolescence is a vulnerable period for cognitive and psychiatric consequences.

Risk Factors for Marijuana Use

The risk for marijuana use begins with the individual and is mediated by familial and cultural factors such as parental disapproval, parental supervision, availability, and perceived risk. Genetic research helps answer questions regarding risk for addiction, and twin studies have been con-

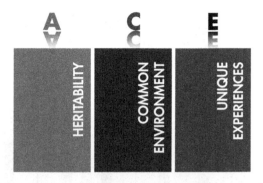

FIGURE 2–5. ACE models of genetic and environmental risks used in twin studies.

Note. A=Additive genetic effects; C=Common environmental effects; E=Environment and experiences unique to each individual.

ducted in which three separate contributions are disentangled. Additive genetic factors are usually denoted "A," shared or common environmental factors denoted "C," and environmental experiences unique to the individual denoted "E" (Figure 2–5). These three factors are measured by determining prevalence rates in fraternal and identical twins relative to the general population. If there is a high concordance between identical twins and a low concordance between fraternal twins, then the condition is thought to be highly genetic and have a high "A." If a condition is equally concordant within sets of identical and fraternal twins, then it is thought to be highly dependent on shared or common environmental "C" factors. If the condition is not well explained by either and concordance between both identical and fraternal twins is very low, then the condition is thought to be driven by unique environmental "E" factors—experiences of one twin and not another. A few of the genes contributing to the common heritable factors are possible to identify, but each gene is usually of low impact to the overall heritable risk. The shared or common environmental and unique environmental factors can also be studied, and childhood sexual abuse in females is a particularly strong unique environmental factor leading to increased likelihood of substance use.

Shared environmental factors often predominate in individuals who initiate use very early because certain factors such as low parental supervision allow genes conferring increased risk taking to manifest in behavior. The ease of access and perceived risk of use are fairly significant for predicting marijuana use. Home environments that help the child understand the risks of marijuana use may actually be reducing the child's risk, and the home en-

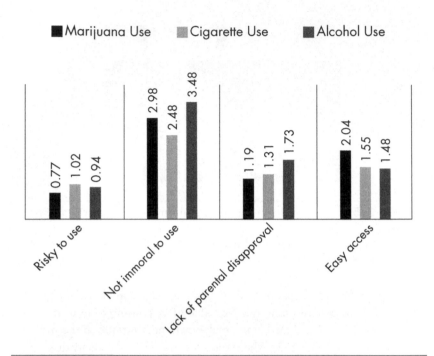

FIGURE 2–6.   Odds ratios for factors related to the onset of use.
Source.   Data from Steen 2010.

vironment that sends the child the message that there is nothing "wrong" with using may be contributing to a threefold elevated risk of use. As shown in Figure 2–6, the specific lack of parental disapproval is associated with modest increases in use (Steen 2010).

A frequent finding from genetically informed studies of substance use is that the shared environment drives initiation of use but that continued and problematic use is driven more by genetic factors. Additive genetic (A), shared environmental (C), and unique environmental (E) effects have been measured for the initiation of marijuana use and the development of marijuana-related problems (Verweij et al. 2010). Beginning to use marijuana was associated with A, C, and E estimates of 40%, 39%, and 21% in females, respectively (Figure 2–7). For the progression to problematic marijuana use, genetics takes over, and the effects of the shared environment are reduced: A, C, and E estimates are 59%, 15%, and 26% for females (Figure 2–8). As seen with other studies, there was a trend for a greater C and lesser A component for initiation of drug use compared with progression to problematic use. This may be because developing marijuana dependence symptoms is more dependent on a biological diathesis than is the decision to begin using,

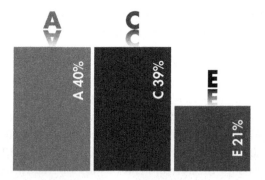

FIGURE 2–7. Marijuana use initiation.
Source. Data from Verweij et al. 2010.

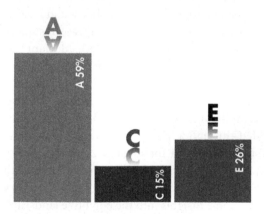

FIGURE 2–8. Progression to problematic marijuana use.
Source. Data from Verweij et al. 2010.

which is more determined by peers, availability, and the influence of shared environmental factors.

For the clinician, figuring out the proportion of risk that is genetically versus environmentally mediated may not be as important in counseling an individual case, but knowing the individual's general level of risk of developing a substance use disorder is important. In Harriet's case, she demonstrated some biobehavioral dysregulation evidenced by picking, impulsively responding, having thought about death, and displaying variable sleep and eating patterns. A measure known as the Transmissible Liability Index (TLI) asks questions about a child's biobehavioral characteristics such as appetite variability, sleep restlessness, picking, oppositionality, and impulsive responding. It uses such questions to measure the transmissible risk for substance use disorders in a given individual by measuring the parental environmentally mediated and genetically mediated risk. The TLI is a highly heritable marker of biologically driven behavioral dysregulation and propensity for social deviance, which thereby reflects an individual's tendency toward developing a substance use disorder (Kirisci et al. 2009). Together with the Non-Transmissible Liability Index (measuring the influence of siblings and extrafamilial factors), it can predict, between the ages of 10 and 12, future cannabis use disorder at age 22 with 75% accuracy (Kirisci et al. 2009). Other constructs, apart from those in the TLI, have been known risk factors for the development of substance use disorders, such as emotional dysregulation and externalizing behaviors. However, the TLI predicts cannabis use disorder risk without these measures, and their inclusion does not add to the predictive model (Kirisci et al. 2015), likely because TLI constructs have encapsulated these factors.

There are powerful effects of nontransmissible liability whereby peers, parental attitudes, neighborhood drug availability, and legal policy all might affect the propensity of a given individual to use substances. There exists some controversy as to whether affiliation with "deviant" peers drives the use of drugs (Tarter et al. 2011) or whether using drugs drives the affiliation with peers who use (Gillespie et al. 2009). The problems are likely bidirectional. Using teens tend to report that their peer group becomes increasingly made up of other individuals who use, but most teens begin using because of access provided through a friend. Whether peer-group deviance is the mechanism or simply a marker for substance use risk, deviant youth are a group greatly in need of preventive interventions to reduce their risk.

Models such as the *reasoned action approach* and the *theory of planned behavior* may provide some insights into the cognitive landscape that is related to drug use (Conner and McMillan 1999). These models try to explain volitional behaviors and thus may be most useful for predicting the initiation of drug use. They are not designed to account for the behaviors that are driven by subconscious processes, such as addictions, but subconscious processes may affect relevant attitudes. In these models, behavioral intention comes from factors termed attitudes toward the behavior, perceived behavioral control, and subjective norms. Attitudes toward the behavior of substance use will vary on the basis of the perceived benefits and the perceived risks. Consistent with the model is the fact that perception of harm is inversely related to heavy use of marijuana in the Monitoring the Future study (Johnston et al. 2014). Important perceived harms related to spontaneous attempts to quit are the perceived impacts of use on health, self-image, and self-control (Chauchard et al. 2013). The expected benefits of using involve the beliefs associated with socialization, intoxication, and, more recently, medical benefits of use. Subjective norms are rapidly changing, and their impact on marijuana use will be important to measure with changes in the legal and cultural landscape.

Examining the presence of psychiatric symptoms that predate marijuana use is difficult because many psychiatric syndromes do not present in childhood but manifest during adolescence or early adulthood. Generally speaking, externalizing syndromes are common precursors to adolescent marijuana use, but internalizing disorders are not (Farmer et al. 2015). Posttraumatic stress disorder (PTSD) has been shown to have a robust association with substance use disorders, and childhood sexual abuse is a durable risk factor for substance use disorders (Cornelius et al. 2010). For individuals with high experiential avoidance (i.e., the tendency to engage in strategies to reduce unpleasant private experiences), higher levels of PTSD symptom severity were associated with a greater risk of cannabis dependence (Bordieri et al. 2014). These examples show an increased risk for substance use driven by the types of traumas satisfying DSM-5 PTSD Criterion A. Coping motives may generate more sympathy from clinicians, but they do not signify a less dangerous trajectory of use. In fact, coping motives have predicted the transition of substance use to dependence (van der Pol et al. 2013), and Buckner et al. (2007) provided evidence that coping motives mediated the association between social phobia and marijuana-related problems.

It is worth mentioning that much of the use of the term *self-medication* goes beyond Khantzian's (1985) original hypothesis that "the drugs that addicts select are not chosen randomly" (p. 1259). Now, lax use of the term has broadened to include all substance use risk driven by psychiatric conditions. Compared with frequent use of the term to explain substance use in individuals with anxiety and depression, the increased rates of substance use by those with conduct disorder do not receive the appellation "self-medicating," but conduct disorder confers a strong risk for marijuana use and marijuana addiction. Conduct disorder mediates most of the increased risk for frequent marijuana use seen in individuals with externalizing disorders (Sibley et al. 2014), but hyperactive-impulsive ADHD symptoms incrementally raise the risk for marijuana use even after controlling for the presence of conduct disorder (Elkins et al. 2007).

Bipolar disorder is a robust predictor of marijuana and other substance use disorders (Compton et al. 2007). Several studies have correlated marijuana use with a worsening course and earlier onset of bipolar disorder (Lagerberg et al. 2011; Strakowski et al. 2007; van Rossum et al. 2009), but the direction of causality is difficult to determine. Genetically informed studies indicate that the overlap of major depression and marijuana use is likely due to shared liabilities, but adolescent-onset marijuana use has been associated with suicidality after controlling for genetic factors (Lynskey et al. 2004; Pedersen 2008). Regardless of the direction of causality, patients with dual diagnosis are in particular need of attention both because it is possible that marijuana use is driving the psychiatric issue (Wittchen et al. 2007) and because marijuana users with comorbid psychiatric disorders are at higher risk of addiction (Lopez-Quintero et al. 2011).

Progression From Marijuana Use to Addiction: Biological Factors and Social Constraints

Whereas DSM-IV cannabis dependence was a binary (i.e., present or absent) disorder, addiction is not a binary condition. DSM-5 better reflects this reality with mild, moderate, and severe specifiers replacing the older abuse-dependence dichotomy, and this more dimensional approach better models the gradual neuroplasticity of the brain in the context of addiction. Whereas the mesolimbic dopamine system may be the first to adapt, changes in other systems continue to develop and overwhelm the individual when an opportunity to use presents itself. Dorsal striatal, and perhaps thalamic, areas adapt to persistent drug exposure, and much of the drug-seeking behavior that was previously motivated and involved the limbic system becomes habitual and rote.

Prefrontal circuitry adaptations lead to deficient inhibition of drug responses. Cortical control of the mesolimbic circuitry malfunctions, and this leads to an overvaluing of drug-related reinforcers and an undervaluing of natural reinforcers. The individual's use gradually becomes more solitary, and his or her range of activities is reduced. Abnormalities in frontocortical regions are associated with decreased impulse control, as well as a preference for immediate rewards over larger, delayed rewards, termed *delay discounting*.

Strengthening of context-dependent associations in the hippocampus may be an important area of neuroplasticity, and one of particular interest for marijuana use progression because the hippocampus is rich in cannabinoid receptors. The extended amygdala also adapts following prolonged use, which leads to a condition of heightened reactivity on discontinuation of a substance, causing craving and dysphoria. Whereas the basolateral amygdala adapts to substance use, the central amygdala likely drives some of the tension and negative emotionality developing later in addiction. The insula is an important area for predicting relapse, and it has been shown that cigarette smokers who suffer strokes to the insula are easily able to quit smoking (Koob and Volkow 2010).

Clinically, these brain phenomena were captured in a 3-year prospective study of the transition from frequent marijuana use to dependence (van der Pol et al. 2013). As previously mentioned, coping motives predicted the transition to dependence, and this may reflect heightened dysphoria seen with neuroplasticity in long-term marijuana use. Living alone, major financial problems, and impaired control over use also predicted transition to dependence over the 3-year course of the study. With continued use, the brain becomes decreasingly responsive to natural reinforcers such as social reward, employment, and companionship. It could be that the association van der Pol and colleagues found between living alone and transitioning to dependence was a reflection of a gradual social withdrawal due to decreased social interest, and that financial problems were reflective of the brain not being as motivated by the pursuit of financial rewards relative to drug reward. All drugs cause a monopolization of motivation toward the drug use, and marijuana may also cause a generalized decrease in motivation beyond other drugs of abuse. Impaired control over use would reflect the mesolimbic and frontal neuroplasticity referenced in Koob and Volkow's (2010) review. Major financial problems might reflect substance-induced executive dysfunction and delay discounting. Whether each of these associations was the result of neuroplastic changes is impossible to say from this study design. Because these factors predicted the transition to dependence among heavy users and variables regarding the individual's actual use pattern (e.g., amount, frequency, potency) were just shy of statistical significance, the results might be misinterpreted to mean that drug exposure and using variables are not important factors in developing cannabis dependence. However, for any given individual, there exists an amount of marijuana-mediated or -driven activity in the brain (moderated by factors such as age at onset) that will drive each neuroplastic change.

The exposure necessary to cross a somewhat artificial threshold for DSM-IV cannabis dependence varies widely among individuals. This variation is due to differences in liabilities among various individuals to meet cannabis dependence criteria. For example, individuals with ample resources may require more substance-driven problems to accumulate enough financial problems to meet criteria of social dysfunction, and individuals with few responsibilities will require a more extensive progression of functional impairment before meeting the criteria of failure to fulfill role obligations. Addiction is a behaviorally defined concept, not a pharmacologically defined one. Intrinsic individual differences also may be important, as some individuals are more likely than others to develop psychological and physical problems following marijuana use.

Although many studies examine the determinants of addiction within a specific culture, it is important to consider cultural variables that could affect the rates of addiction. Variable social constraints on the use of marijuana emerge through one's 20s because it becomes less socially acceptable to engage in illicit drug use in professional careers and many employers are screening for substance use. Also, there are perhaps *practical* constraints of regular marijuana use that emerge during early adulthood as the difficulties marijuana can cause with memory and occupational functioning lead people to voluntarily discontinue use.

Removing social constraints on use of a drug (i.e., decriminalization and legalization) because it has a lower rate of addiction may be removing the very thing that causes that lower rate of addiction. As has been pointed out, "The effects of a drug (legal or illegal) on individual health are determined not only by its pharmacologic properties but also by its availability and social acceptability. In this respect, legal drugs (alcohol and tobacco) offer a sobering perspective, accounting for the greatest burden of disease associated with drugs not because they are more dangerous than illegal drugs but because their legal status allows for more widespread exposure" (Volkow et al. 2014a, pp. 2225–2226).

Marijuana Dependence and Withdrawal

Members of the lay public often ask whether marijuana is "physically addictive" or "just psychologically addictive." *Physical addiction* and *psychological addiction* are not technical terms; every addiction has a physical reality evidenced by known involvement of structures such as the VTA, nucleus accumbens, prefrontal cortex, anterior cingulate, amygdala, insula, hippocampus, and other brain regions. Most people using the terms physical and psychological dependence or addiction in this context are referring to the question of whether the body can experience withdrawal on cessation of marijuana use. The science is unequivocal and led to the inclusion of cannabis withdrawal in DSM-5. Clinical laboratory measures and information gathered from clinical interviews validate the syndrome of marijuana withdrawal. Cessation of marijuana use involves the development of a withdrawal syndrome that includes irritability, aggression, anxiety, sleep difficulty, decreased appetite, restlessness, dysphoria, abdominal pain, shakiness, sweating, fever, chills, and headache (Budney et al. 2004). Because individuals frequently use nicotine and marijuana together and may stop using both at the same time, the withdrawal syndromes commonly co-occur. However, marijuana withdrawal symptoms do not completely overlap with symptoms of nicotine withdrawal, allowing them to be differentiated. Overall, the two conditions have similar withdrawal severity, but there are large differences between individuals regarding which substance affects them more severely. Some individuals experience more impairment from nicotine withdrawal, and some experience more impairment from marijuana withdrawal (Vandrey et al. 2008).

The physically addictive properties of marijuana, more properly termed *pharmacological dependence,* play a role in the maintenance of addiction. Marijuana withdrawal symptoms have a negative correlation with successful substance abuse treatment outcomes; greater functional impairment from marijuana withdrawal symptoms is associated with relapses to marijuana after abstinence (Allsop et al. 2012). Ecological momentary analysis, which tracks an individual's moods and motivations throughout the day, shows that withdrawal symptoms on a given day predict greater marijuana use at later time points throughout the day (Buckner et al. 2015).

Beyond increased risk for relapse, the withdrawal syndrome is associated with increased frequency of violent and aggressive behavior in clinical laboratory settings. That is, in clinical laboratory studies of withdrawal, aggression is frequently seen (Budney et al. 2003) and is an important factor for clinicians to consider in recently abstinent marijuana users.

Although ICD-10 (World Health Organization 1992) does not allow for coding cannabis withdrawal in the setting of mild substance use disorder, studies indicate that withdrawal may occur. An individual does not have to be using for years, or even have a DSM diagnosis of a cannabis use disorder, to develop the syndrome; a study of treatment-seeking adolescents and young adults found common marijuana withdrawal symptoms on cessation: craving (82%), irritability (76%), restlessness (58%), anxiety (55%), and depression (52%) (Cornelius et al. 2008).

Marijuana's Effects on Development

Marijuana use during pregnancy can lead to neurophysiological and behavioral abnormalities in the offspring, and animal research has demonstrated causal mechanisms of intrauterine marijuana exposure that might explain the associations seen in human studies (Calvigioni et al. 2014). Many of these effects are due to THC disrupting neurons in the developing human brain, growing from deep in the brain, finding their way to the proper location in higher brain areas, selecting targets for synapse formation, and forming those synapses (Berghuis et al. 2007). Prenatal marijuana exposure has been shown to have enduring effects in a variety of outcomes through animal studies (Spano et al. 2010), and there are associations found in human studies with social, cognitive, and motor functioning (Fried and Smith 2001). Specifically, executive dysfunction is one of the common effects thought to occur from intrauterine exposure. Preclinical data suggest there could be substantial developmental effects because cannabinoid receptors are transiently expressed in many brain areas prenatally and postnatally (Gaffuri et al. 2012). Prenatal marijuana exposure predicts adolescent and young adult marijuana use after controlling for exposure to other drugs, family history of substance use disorder, parental strictness or supervision, delinquency, and other factors (Sonon et al. 2015).

Because the prefrontal cortex is undergoing active development from early childhood through adolescence, it is reasonable to assume that the sensitive period documented in adolescence extends at least partially to childhood. The effects of THC in animal models of the prenatal and adolescent periods are well known (Calvigioni et al. 2014; Dinieri and Hurd 2012), but the effects on early childhood are not well studied.

The effects of THC on gender development are also likely to be substantial because estrogen's effects on the development of the female nervous system depend on well-regulated functioning of the endocannabinoid system (Karasu et al. 2011). Aspects of female development regulated by the central nervous system, including maternal-fetal interactions and the release of hormones that affect the rest of the body, may be disrupted by the presence of THC.

Adolescent marijuana exposure has developmentally sensitive critical effects on processes such as synaptic pruning (Malone et al. 2010) and axonal pathfinding (Zalesky et al. 2012). The potentially disruptive effects on the prefrontal cortex due to THC exposure during adolescence are an area of great concern (Bossong and Niesink 2010). Adolescent exposure has been associated with deficits in a wide variety of cognitive tasks (Randolph et al. 2013). As mentioned earlier, the effects of THC use by adolescents on IQ seem to be permanent: a loss of 5–8 IQ points (Meier et al. 2012), or the same amount of intellectual impairment seen in children who are exposed to high levels (10 µg/dL) of lead (Canfield et al. 2003).

Key Points

- Mental health professionals should take into account the acute and chronic effects of marijuana use when assessing the needs of patients presenting with psychiatric symptoms.
- The mechanisms underlying the addictive properties of marijuana are similar to those underlying the addictive properties of all other drugs of abuse, and marijuana use leads to alterations in motivated behavior. Beyond this, there is some evidence that actions on the cannabinoid receptors outside of the mesolimbic system affect motivation.
- Marijuana's effects on cognition and motivation may contribute to deficits in psychosocial functioning. The effects of adolescent use are clinically significant and are thought to persist following cessation.
- There are known risk factors for substance use disorders. Early-onset use, family history, posttraumatic stress disorder, and externalizing disorders are associated with increased risk of marijuana use and addiction.
- Marijuana use is associated with the development of acute psychotic, mood, and anxiety symptoms that may be the cause of clinical attention.
- The effects of marijuana on the brain depend on the developmental stage of the individual.

References

Agrawal A, Neale MC, Prescott CA, et al: A twin study of early cannabis use and subsequent use and abuse/dependence of other illicit drugs. Psychol Med 34(7):1227–1237, 2004 15697049

Albrecht DS, Skosnik PD, Vollmer JM, et al: Striatal D(2)/D(3) receptor availability is inversely correlated with cannabis consumption in chronic marijuana users. Drug Alcohol Depend 128(1–2):52–57, 2013 22909787

Allsop DJ, Copeland J, Norberg MM, et al: Quantifying the clinical significance of cannabis withdrawal. PLoS One 7(9):e44864, 2012 23049760

American Psychiatric Association: Diagnostic and Statistical Manual of Mental Disorders, 4th Edition. Washington, DC, American Psychiatric Association, 1994

American Psychiatric Association: Diagnostic and Statistical Manual of Mental Disorders, 5th Edition. Arlington, VA, American Psychiatric Association, 2013

Behrendt S, Wittchen HU, Höfler M, et al: Transitions from first substance use to substance use disorders in adolescence: is early onset associated with a rapid escalation? Drug Alcohol Depend 99(1–3):68–78, 2009 18768267

Berghuis P, Rajnicek AM, Morozov YM, et al: Hardwiring the brain: endocannabinoids shape neuronal connectivity. Science 316(5828):1212–1216, 2007 17525344

Bolla KI, Lesage SR, Gamaldo CE, et al: Polysomnogram changes in marijuana users who report sleep disturbances during prior abstinence. Sleep Med 11(9):882–889, 2010 20685163

Bordieri MJ, Tull MT, McDermott MJ, et al: The moderating role of experiential avoidance in the relationship between posttraumatic stress disorder symptom severity and cannabis dependence. J Contextual Behav Sci 3(4):273–278, 2014 25478317

Bossong MG, Niesink RJ: Adolescent brain maturation, the endogenous cannabinoid system and the neurobiology of cannabis-induced schizophrenia. Prog Neurobiol 92(3):370–385, 2010 20624444

Brook JS, Stimmel MA, Zhang C, et al: The association between earlier marijuana use and subsequent academic achievement and health problems: a longitudinal study. Am J Addict 17(2):155–160, 2008 18393060

Buckner JD, Bonn-Miller MO, Zvolensky MJ, et al: Marijuana use motives and social anxiety among marijuana-using young adults. Addict Behav 32(10):2238–2252, 2007 17478056

Buckner JD, Zvolensky MJ, Crosby RD, et al: Antecedents and consequences of cannabis use among racially diverse cannabis users: an analysis from Ecological Momentary Assessment. Drug Alcohol Depend 147:20–25, 2015 25578250

Budney AJ, Moore BA, Vandrey RG, et al: The time course and significance of cannabis withdrawal. J Abnorm Psychol 112(3):393–402, 2003 12943018

Budney AJ, Hughes JR, Moore BA, et al: Review of the validity and significance of cannabis withdrawal syndrome. Am J Psychiatry 161(11):1967–1977, 2004 15514394

Budney AJ, Roffman R, Stephens RS, et al: Marijuana dependence and its treatment. Addict Sci Clin Pract 4(1):4–16, 2007 18292704

Calvigioni D, Hurd YL, Harkany T, et al: Neuronal substrates and functional consequences of prenatal cannabis exposure. Eur Child Adolesc Psychiatry 23(10):931–941, 2014 24793873

Canfield RL, Henderson CR Jr, Cory-Slechta DA, et al: Intellectual impairment in children with blood lead concentrations below 10 microg per deciliter. N Engl J Med 348(16):1517–1526, 2003 12700371

Casey BJ, Jones RM: Neurobiology of the adolescent brain and behavior: implications for substance use disorders. J Am Acad Child Adolesc Psychiatry 49(12):1189–1201, quiz 1285, 2010 21093769

Chauchard E, Levin KH, Copersino ML, et al: Motivations to quit cannabis use in an adult non-treatment sample: are they related to relapse? Addict Behav 38(9):2422–2427, 2013 23685328

Compton WM, Thomas YF, Stinson FS, et al: Prevalence, correlates, disability, and comorbidity of DSM-IV drug abuse and dependence in the United States: results from the National Epidemiologic Survey on Alcohol and Related Conditions. Arch Gen Psychiatry 64(5):566–576, 2007 17485608

Conner M, McMillan B: Interaction effects in the theory of planned behaviour: studying cannabis use. Br J Soc Psychol 38 (Pt 2):195–222, 1999 10392450

Cooper ZD, Haney M: Cannabis reinforcement and dependence: role of the cannabinoid CB1 receptor. Addict Biol 13(2):188–195, 2008 18279497

Cornelius JR, Chung T, Martin C, et al: Cannabis withdrawal is common among treatment-seeking adolescents with cannabis dependence and major depression, and is associated with rapid relapse to dependence. Addict Behav 33(11):1500–1505, 2008 18313860

Cornelius JR, Kirisci L, Reynolds M, et al: PTSD contributes to teen and young adult cannabis use disorders. Addict Behav 35(2):91–94, 2010 19773127

Degenhardt L, Coffey C, Romaniuk H, et al: The persistence of the association between adolescent cannabis use and common mental disorders into young adulthood. Addiction 108(1):124–133, 2013 22775447

Dinieri JA, Hurd YL: Rat models of prenatal and adolescent cannabis exposure. Methods Mol Biol 829:231–242, 2012 22231817

Elkins IJ, McGue M, Iacono WG: Prospective effects of attention-deficit/hyperactivity disorder, conduct disorder, and sex on adolescent substance use and abuse. Arch Gen Psychiatry 64(10):1145–1152, 2007 17909126

Farmer RF, Seeley JR, Kosty DB, et al: Internalizing and externalizing psychopathology as predictors of cannabis use disorder onset during adolescence and early adulthood. Psychol Addict Behav 29(3):541–551, 2015 25799438

Fontes MA, Bolla KI, Cunha PJ, et al: Cannabis use before age 15 and subsequent executive functioning. Br J Psychiatry 198(6):442–447, 2011 21628706

Fried PA, Smith AM: A literature review of the consequences of prenatal marihuana exposure: an emerging theme of a deficiency in aspects of executive function. Neurotoxicol Teratol 23(1):1–11, 2001 11274871

Gaffuri AL, Ladarre D, Lenkei Z: Type-1 cannabinoid receptor signaling in neuronal development. Pharmacology 90(1–2):19–39, 2012 22776780

Gillespie NA, Neale MC, Jacobson K, et al: Modeling the genetic and environmental association between peer group deviance and cannabis use in male twins. Addiction 104(3):420–429, 2009 19207350

Grant JD, Lynskey MT, Scherrer JF, et al: A cotwin-control analysis of drug use and abuse/dependence risk associated with early onset cannabis use. Addict Behav 35(1):35–41, 2010 19717242

Grant JE, Chamberlain SR, Schreiber L, et al: Neuropsychological deficits associated with cannabis use in young adults. Drug Alcohol Depend 121(1–2):159–162, 2012 21920674

Hall W: What has research over the past two decades revealed about the adverse health effects of recreational cannabis use? Addiction 110(1):19–35, 2015 25287883

Hurd YL, Michaelides M, Miller ML, et al: Trajectory of adolescent cannabis use on addiction vulnerability. Neuropharmacology 76 (Pt B):416–424, 2014 23954491

Iversen LL: The Science of Marijuana, 2nd Edition. New York, Oxford University Press, 2008

Johnston LD, O'Malley PM, Miech RA: Monitoring the Future: National Survey Results on Drug Use, 1975–2013—Overview, Key Findings on Adolescent Drug Use. Ann Arbor, University of Michigan, 2014

Karasu T, Marczylo TH, Maccarrone M, et al: The role of sex steroid hormones, cytokines and the endocannabinoid system in female fertility. Hum Reprod Update 17(3):347–361, 2011 21227997

Khan SS, Secades-Villa R, Okuda M, et al: Gender differences in cannabis use disorders: results from the National Epidemiologic Survey of Alcohol and Related Conditions. Drug Alcohol Depend 130(1–3):101–108, 2013 23182839

Khani A, Kermani M, Hesam S, et al: Activation of cannabinoid system in anterior cingulate cortex and orbitofrontal cortex modulates cost-benefit decision making. Psychopharmacology (Berl) 232(12):2097–2112, 2015 25529106

Khantzian EJ: The self-medication hypothesis of addictive disorders: focus on heroin and cocaine dependence. Am J Psychiatry 142(11):1259–1264, 1985 3904487

Kirisci L, Tarter R, Mezzich A, et al: Prediction of cannabis use disorder between boyhood and young adulthood: clarifying the phenotype and environtype. Am J Addict 18(1):36–47, 2009 19219664

Kirisci L, Tarter R, Ridenour T, et al: Externalizing behavior and emotion dysregulation are indicators of transmissible risk for substance use disorder. Addict Behav 42:57–62, 2015 25462655

Koob GF, Volkow ND: Neurocircuitry of addiction. Neuropsychopharmacology 35(1):217–238, 2010 19710631

Kowal MA, Hazekamp A, Colzato LS, et al: Cannabis and creativity: highly potent cannabis impairs divergent thinking in regular cannabis users. Psychopharmacology (Berl) 232(6):1123–1134, 2015 25288512

Lagerberg TV, Sundet K, Aminoff SR, et al: Excessive cannabis use is associated with earlier age at onset in bipolar disorder. Eur Arch Psychiatry Clin Neurosci 261(6):397–405, 2011 21267743

Lopez-Quintero C, Pérez de los Cobos J, Hasin DS, et al: Probability and predictors of transition from first use to dependence on nicotine, alcohol, cannabis, and cocaine: results of the National Epidemiologic Survey on Alcohol and Related Conditions (NESARC). Drug Alcohol Depend 115(1–2):120–130, 2011 21145178

Lynskey MT, Heath AC, Bucholz KK, et al: Escalation of drug use in early onset cannabis users vs co-twin controls. JAMA 289(4):427–433, 2003 12533121

Lynskey MT, Glowinski AL, Todorov AA, et al: Major depressive disorder, suicidal ideation, and suicide attempt in twins discordant for cannabis dependence and early onset cannabis use. Arch Gen Psychiatry 61(10):1026–1032, 2004 15466676

Malone DT, Hill MN, Rubino T: Adolescent cannabis use and psychosis: epidemiology and neurodevelopmental models. Br J Pharmacol 160(3):511–522, 2010 20590561

McDonald J, Schleifer L, Richards JB, et al: Effects of THC on behavioral measures of impulsivity in humans. Neuropsychopharmacology 28(7):1356–1365, 2003 12784123

Meier MH, Caspi A, Ambler A, et al: Persistent cannabis users show neuropsychological decline from childhood to midlife. Proc Natl Acad Sci USA 109(40):E2657–E2664, 2012 22927402

Moffitt TE, Meier MH, Caspi A, et al: Reply to Rogeberg and Daly: No evidence that socioeconomic status or personality differences confound the association between cannabis use and IQ decline. Proc Natl Acad Sci USA 110(11):E980–E982, 2013 23599952

Palamar JJ, Fenstermaker M, Kamboukos D, et al: Adverse psychosocial outcomes associated with drug use among US high school seniors: a comparison of alcohol and marijuana. Am J Drug Alcohol Abuse 40(6):438–446, 2014 25169838

Pedersen W: Does cannabis use lead to depression and suicidal behaviours? A population-based longitudinal study. Acta Psychiatr Scand 118(5):395–403, 2008 18798834

Randolph K, Turull P, Margolis A, et al: Cannabis and cognitive systems in adolescents. Adolesc Psychiatry 3(2):135–147, 2013

Sibley MH, Pelham WE, Molina BS, et al: The role of early childhood ADHD and subsequent CD in the initiation and escalation of adolescent cigarette, alcohol, and marijuana use. J Abnorm Psychol 123(2):362–374, 2014 24886010

Solowij N, Jones KA, Rozman ME, et al: Reflection impulsivity in adolescent cannabis users: a comparison with alcohol-using and non-substance-using adolescents. Psychopharmacology (Berl) 219(2):575–586, 2012 21938415

Sonon KE, Richardson GA, Cornelius JR, et al: Prenatal marijuana exposure predicts marijuana use in young adulthood. Neurotoxicol Teratol 47:10–15, 2015 25446014

Spano MS, Fadda P, Fratta W, et al: Cannabinoid-opioid interactions in drug discrimination and self-administration: effect of maternal, postnatal, adolescent and adult exposure to the drugs. Curr Drug Targets 11(4):450–461, 2010 20017729

Steen JA: A multilevel study of the role of environment in adolescent substance use. J Child Adolesc Subst Abuse 19(5):359–371, 2010

Strakowski SM, DelBello MP, Fleck DE, et al: Effects of co-occurring cannabis use disorders on the course of bipolar disorder after a first hospitalization for mania. Arch Gen Psychiatry 64(1):57–64, 2007 17199055

Swift W, Coffey C, Carlin JB, et al: Adolescent cannabis users at 24 years: trajectories to regular weekly use and dependence in young adulthood. Addiction 103(8):1361–1370, 2008 18855826

Swift W, Coffey C, Carlin JB, et al: Are adolescents who moderate their cannabis use at lower risk of later regular and dependent cannabis use? Addiction 104(5):806–814, 2009 19344439

Tarter RE, Fishbein D, Kirisci L, et al: Deviant socialization mediates transmissible and contextual risk on cannabis use disorder development: a prospective study. Addiction 106(7):1301–1308, 2011 21320228

Thames AD, Arbid N, Sayegh P: Cannabis use and neurocognitive functioning in a non-clinical sample of users. Addict Behav 39(5):994–999, 2014 24556155

van der Pol P, Liebregts N, de Graaf R, et al: Predicting the transition from frequent cannabis use to cannabis dependence: a three-year prospective study. Drug Alcohol Depend 133(2):352–359, 2013 23886472

Vandrey RG, Budney AJ, Hughes JR, et al: A within-subject comparison of withdrawal symptoms during abstinence from cannabis, tobacco, and both substances. Drug Alcohol Depend 92(1–3):48–54, 2008 17643868

van Rossum I, Boomsma M, Tenback D, et al: Does cannabis use affect treatment outcome in bipolar disorder? A longitudinal analysis. J Nerv Ment Dis 197(1):35–40, 2009 19155808

Verweij KJ, Zietsch BP, Lynskey MT, et al: Genetic and environmental influences on cannabis use initiation and problematic use: a meta-analysis of twin studies. Addiction 105(3):417–430, 2010 20402985

Volkow ND, Fowler JS, Wang GJ, et al: Dopamine in drug abuse and addiction: results from imaging studies and treatment implications. Mol Psychiatry 9(6):557–569, 2004 15098002

Volkow ND, Wang GJ, Fowler JS, et al: Addiction: decreased reward sensitivity and increased expectation sensitivity conspire to overwhelm the brain's control circuit. Bioessays 32(9):748–755, 2010 20730946

Volkow ND, Baler RD, Compton WM, et al: Adverse health effects of marijuana use. N Engl J Med 370(23):2219–2227, 2014a 24897085

Volkow ND, Wang GJ, Telang F, et al: Decreased dopamine brain reactivity in marijuana abusers is associated with negative emotionality and addiction severity. Proc Natl Acad Sci USA 111(30):E3149–E3156, 2014b 25024177

Wittchen HU, Fröhlich C, Behrendt S, et al: Cannabis use and cannabis use disorders and their relationship to mental disorders: a 10-year prospective-longitudinal community study in adolescents. Drug Alcohol Depend 88 (suppl 1):S60–S70, 2007 17257779

World Health Organization: International Classification of Diseases, 10th Revision. Geneva, World Health Organization, 1992

Zalesky A, Solowij N, Yücel M, et al: Effect of long-term cannabis use on axonal fibre connectivity. Brain 135 (Pt 7):2245–2255, 2012 22669080

CHAPTER 3

Medical and Recreational Marijuana Policy

From Prohibition to the Rise of Legalization

Arthur Robin Williams, M.D., M.B.E.

Clinical Vignette: Marcus Requests a "Prescription for Medical Marijuana"

Marcus Jones is a 32-year-old single, employed male who has been coming to a mental health clinic for the past few months for treatment of dysthymia and is now taking escitalopram 20 mg daily with moderate benefit. Recently, he has been increasingly bothered by anxiety and initial insomnia, and he requests a "prescription for medical marijuana" after hearing from a friend that it works "better and faster" than antidepressant or anxiolytic medications. The state in which the clinic is located approved a medical marijuana program a few years ago, but the staff psychiatrist, Dr. Marvin Stein, is not sure if anxiety is an indication for enrollment and is worried about medicolegal liability. Dr. Stein explains these concerns to Marcus, but Marcus gets frustrated and says, "Fine, then I'll just go to Colorado and buy some without your help."

The author wishes to acknowledge the helpful feedback provided by Mark Olfson, M.D., M.P.H.

This case raises a number of questions. What is the physician's role in the evaluation and care of patients seeking medical marijuana? Are there any psychiatric indications for medical marijuana? How do medical marijuana programs differ across states? How do states that have legalized marijuana differ from those with medical marijuana programs alone? What are the implications for mental health providers if their patients use "legal" marijuana?

Overview of Drug Control Policy

Legal access to marijuana has changed dramatically over the past 20 years in the United States. Generally speaking, these changes have involved reforms at the state level. In order to understand the sometimes very nuanced distinctions between states' approaches to marijuana access, and implications for effects at the population level, this chapter will begin with a review of concepts underlying approaches to general drug control policy, including 1) supply reduction versus demand reduction, 2) substitution versus complement distinctions, and 3) differences between models of decriminalization versus full commercial legalization.

The current approach to drug control policy in the United States largely stems from the "War on Drugs" dating from the early 1970s during the Nixon administration. Although the War on Drugs has become synonymous with harsh penalties and a criminal justice approach to all matters of drug production, sales, and possession, early priorities emphasized treatment and prevention. In fact, the early years of the War on Drugs saw close to 80% of federal funding dedicated to "demand" reduction through treatment and prevention campaigns (Baum 1997). During the 1980s and 1990s, however, it became politically expedient to emphasize "supply" reduction through interdiction and law enforcement efforts to disrupt supply chains (Strang et al. 2012). There are differing views about which approach works best, although there is growing consensus that the widespread use of intoxicating substances and black market activity have persisted despite decades of intense supply reduction approaches and mass incarceration.

Each drug of abuse, such as marijuana, theoretically has its own demand curve related to the population's perception of harm related to its use; the cost of use, including price as well as the effort needed to obtain the drug; and the legal risks of obtaining and possessing the drug (Caulkins et al. 2012a). In general, as drugs become cheaper and more available, rates of use increase. Like other market goods, the price elasticity of demand for a given drug affects its consumption (Nordstrom and Kleber 2011). *Price elasticity* refers to the percent change in consumption of a given good divided by the percent change in price. The consumption of goods that are unnecessary (such has gourmet chocolate) tends to be more price-sensitive, whereas staples (such as bread and toilet paper) tend to be price-inelastic. For instance, the increasing cost of cigarettes led to greater declines in use among younger adults in part as a result of greater price elasticity of demand among the young adult market.

Part of what affects the price elasticity of and overall demand for a drug is how the drug may serve as a complement to or substitute for similar products. For instance, convincing arguments can be made for marijuana and alcohol either as complements or as substitutes (Anderson and Rees 2014). Pro-legalization advocates suggest that increased use of marijuana will lead to decreased consumption of alcohol because marijuana is a substitute good. Indeed, some analyses suggest that alcohol-related traffic fatalities dropped around 10% following the implementation of medical marijuana laws (Anderson and Rees 2011). Some studies, however, have found that states with medical marijuana programs may experience increases in alcohol consumption by some individuals because heavy drinking and binge-drinking behaviors can be complementary to marijuana use and are positively associated in epidemiological studies (Anderson and Rees 2014; Choi 2014).

Marijuana pro-legalization advocates often discuss ending prohibition without providing many details about what regime should follow (Caulkins et al. 2012a). Although the discussion of the legal status of marijuana is often reduced to three options (full prohibition, decriminalization, or legalization), according to drug historian David Courtwright (2002), there are at least seven significant regulatory categories for psychoactive drugs:

1. *Pure prohibition:* no manufacture, sale, or use allowed (e.g., heroin)
2. *Prohibitory prescription:* administered directly by physicians for narrow therapeutic purposes (e.g., cocaine)
3. *Maintenance:* supervised prescription allowed for addiction treatment (e.g., methadone)
4. *Regulatory prescription:* use allowed with valid prescriptions only (e.g., oxycodone)
5. *Restricted adult access:* legal limitations on adult access (e.g., alcohol, and marijuana in four states at the time of this writing)
6. *Unrestricted adult access:* adult status as the only requirement for access (e.g., tobacco)
7. *Universal access:* available to anyone (e.g., caffeine)

Under this model, decriminalization is akin to restricted adult access (number 5 above), and legalization is most similar to unrestricted adult access (number 6 above); however, there are many models of decriminalization and legalization that can be put in place. Between 2012 and 2015, four states began to implement regimes for legalizing marijuana (regulating all steps "from seed to sale") in the United States, with varying approaches that may ultimately affect the demand curve within their states, as discussed in more detail later in this chapter.

Marijuana Policy: A Brief Modern History

Early Marijuana Laws

Until the early twentieth century, drug control laws restricting access to intoxicants were entirely left up to the states (ending with the Harrison Narcotics Tax Act of 1914) and were often the by-product of racial and xenophobic animus (Musto 1999; National Commission on Marihuana and Drug Abuse 1972). Similar to the promulgation of laws prohibiting opium, which targeted Chinese immigrants in the late 1800s, municipalities and states began to pass bans on marijuana following the influx of Mexican immigrants escaping the Mexican Revolution (Barcott 2015). California was the first state to outlaw marijuana, in 1913, and other states in the West and Deep South soon followed suit, so that by the early 1930s most states had prohibited the drug (National Commission on Marihuana and Drug Abuse 1972).

Marijuana prohibition arose on a national scale with the passage of the Marihuana Tax Act of 1937, superseding all state-level laws (Table 3–1). Although the federal government had regulated the clear labeling of cannabis-based tinctures and pharmaceuticals under the Pure Food and Drug Act of 1906, effectively creating what is now the U.S. Food and Drug Administration (FDA), it did not attempt to restrict access to marijuana until the Marihuana Tax Act.

Building on the model of the 1914 Harrison Narcotics Tax Act, which taxed the sale of narcotics (any compound related to opium or cocaine) by registered pharmacists (and effectively criminalized unregistered and untaxed sales), the Marihuana Tax Act levied a $1 per ounce tax on registered sales, such as sales by pharmacists to patients who had a valid prescription from a physician, versus a $100 per ounce penalty on unregistered or black market sales (the rough equivalent of an astronomical 700% tax rate in inflation-adjusted dollars) (Barcott 2015). Historian David Musto (1999) notes, however, that by the time the act was passed in 1937, the regulations on physician prescription of marijuana "were so complicated that they [were] not likely to have prescribed it" (p. 91). Nonetheless, the new law criminalized sales of marijuana between individuals. Following the Marihuana Tax Act, law enforcement officials began to criminally prosecute Americans nationwide for selling and possessing marijuana.

TABLE 3–1. Timeline of marijuana-related laws and major pertinent historical events

Event	Year	Significance
Pure Food and Drug Act	1906	Created a role for the federal regulation of product labeling of commonly used substances to prevent the manufacture, sale, or transportation of adulterated, misbranded, or harmful food and drugs. Prior to the law, consumers often bought pharmaceuticals over the counter with unknown amounts of narcotics and adulterants.
Harrison Narcotics Tax Act	1914	Required physicians prescribing narcotics (opium or cocaine derivatives) to register annually with the federal government. Although it did not apply to marijuana, the Harrison Act became the model for drug regulation (e.g., prohibition) on the federal level.
Marihuana Tax Act	1937	The federal government's first attempt at effectively prohibiting marijuana. The act imposed strict registration and reporting requirements and astronomical taxes on recreational marijuana.
United Nations Single Convention on Narcotic Drugs	1961	The United States advocated for worldwide drug prohibition by encouraging developed nations to commit to adopting any measures necessary to prevent the misuse of and illicit trafficking of all drugs of abuse, including marijuana.
Federally licensed marijuana cultivation	1968	The University of Mississippi was contracted under the DEA as the sole source of marijuana for government use, such as NIH-funded research activities.
Controlled Substances Act	1970	Passed as part of the Comprehensive Drug Abuse Prevention and Control Act. The CSA created the scheduling system for addictive substances and led to the classification of marijuana under the DEA and FDA as a Schedule I substance, meaning that it has no therapeutic value and has high potential for harm.
Beginning of the "War on Drugs"	1971	President Nixon declared, "America's public enemy number one in the U.S. is drug abuse. In order to fight and defeat this enemy, it is necessary to wage a new, all-out offensive," initiating what is colloquially referred to as the "War on Drugs."

TABLE 3–1.　Timeline of marijuana-related laws and major pertinent historical events *(continued)*

Event	Year	Significance
First medical marijuana program	1996	California voters passed Proposition 215 to protect the legal rights of patients and their caregivers in possession of marijuana for medical purposes with a physician's recommendation.
Gonzales v. Raich (U.S. Supreme Court)	2005	In a six-to-three opinion delivered by Justice John Paul Stevens, the Court held that the commerce clause gives Congress authority to prohibit the local cultivation and use of marijuana, despite state laws to the contrary.
Ogden memo	2009	U.S. Deputy Attorney General David Ogden released a memo that the Department of Justice will not target "individuals whose actions are in clear and unambiguous compliance with existing state laws providing for the medical use of marijuana," leading state legislatures to expand licensed production of and dispensaries for medical marijuana.
State legalization of recreational marijuana	2012	In November 2012, voters in Washington State and Colorado passed amendments to allow recreational production, sales, and possession of marijuana by adults over the age of 21 years. Alaska, Oregon, and the District of Columbia joined them in 2014.

Note.　CSA=Controlled Substances Act; DEA=U.S. Drug Enforcement Administration; FDA=U.S. Food and Drug Administration; NIH=National Institutes of Health.

Modern Marijuana Drug Control

The practice of criminalizing marijuana sales and possession could have come to an abrupt halt with a mostly forgotten U.S. Supreme Court ruling involving Timothy Leary, a psychedelic guru and 1960s cultural figure, in the spring of 1969. The high court unanimously invalidated the Marihuana Tax Act on the grounds that the requirement of registration was a form of self-incrimination and was unconstitutional according to the Fifth Amendment. In response, President Richard Nixon, known for a strong law enforcement platform, worked with Congress to pass the Controlled Substances Act (CSA) in 1970. The CSA was part of the broader Comprehensive Drug Abuse Prevention and Control Act, which created the scheduling system under the direction of the

U.S. attorney general for what are now known as controlled substances (see Table 3–1). As a result, marijuana was classified as a Schedule I substance, meaning that it has no accepted medical uses and a high potential for abuse.

Current controversy over the classification of marijuana as a Schedule I substance overshadows the contentious process by which marijuana was originally scheduled. The CSA led to the creation of a presidential commission on marijuana to advise the U.S. attorney general on how to classify marijuana. The resulting product, the Shafer Commission Report (National Commission on Marihuana and Drug Abuse 1972), was compiled under the guidance of former Pennsylvania governor Raymond Shafer, a lifelong Republican handpicked by President Nixon (Barcott 2015). To the dismay of the president, the Shafer Commission ultimately produced a report titled *Marihuana: A Signal of Misunderstanding,* largely debunking the *Reefer Madness* propaganda of the prior decades. Although the report proved insufficient to deter the classification of marijuana as a Schedule I drug, it inspired almost a dozen states (Alaska, California, Colorado, Maine, Michigan, Minnesota, New York, North Carolina, Ohio, and Oregon) over the succeeding decade to decriminalize possession of small amounts of marijuana and renewed interest in the potential medicinal applications of marijuana.

In fact, the growing consensus in the 1970s was that the repeal of marijuana prohibition was inevitable with the election of President Jimmy Carter, who was known to have favored civil fines over prison sentences for simple marijuana possession (Barcott 2015). However, because of a conflagration of scandals involving President Carter's drug czar and parent activism driven by worry about teen access to marijuana, the repeal of prohibition never came to pass (Baum 1997). Rather than penalties for marijuana being softened, the 1980s and 1990s witnessed the expansion of draconian drug control laws enhancing mandatory minimum sentences, "three strikes" laws, and mass incarceration. By the end of the century, almost a million arrests were being made every year for marijuana-related offenses (Federal Bureau of Investigation 2001).

Medical Marijuana

Symbolic Reform

Medical marijuana programs were initially promoted as compassionate care programs for severely and terminally ill patients whose illnesses had not responded to conventional treatments. Typically, they were meant to protect the rights of patients using marijuana to treat symptoms such as nausea, cachexia, or spasticity (Hill 2015b). Between 1979 and 1991, five states—Virginia (1979), New Hampshire (1981), Connecticut (1981), Wisconsin (1988), and

Louisiana (1991)—passed laws that legalized medical marijuana with a physician's "prescription." However, these laws were considered symbolic because federal law prohibits physicians from prescribing marijuana given its status as a Schedule I drug.

Medical Marijuana Programs

Medical orientation. More recently, as of the time of this writing, beginning with California in 1996, 23 states (and the District of Columbia) have authorized legal protections for the possession of marijuana for medicinal purposes or have gone even further to create state agencies to license the production, manufacturing, and dispensation of medical marijuana and derivative products (Figure 3–1).

States vary greatly in the requirements and provisions allowable under their medical marijuana laws (Pacula and Sevigny 2014). Although physicians have rarely been involved in crafting medical marijuana laws or regulations for resultant medical marijuana programs, they are tasked in all participating states with "recommending" the use of marijuana to eligible individuals, who then commonly seek registration in a medical marijuana program (Sevigny et al. 2014). More than one million Americans were estimated to be participating in the 19 medical marijuana programs operating as of October 2014 (ProCon.org 2015).

In many states, individuals receive recommendations for marijuana from physicians whom they have seen for a single visit, from whom they receive no diagnosis, and with whom they do not follow up for ongoing care (Song 2010). Yet very little research has assessed how medical marijuana program policies vary across states with respect to basic tenets of medical practice and pharmaceutical regulation (Sevigny et al. 2014; Wilkinson and D'Souza 2014).

Considerable variation exists in the medical orientation of medical marijuana programs. Although just over half of medical marijuana programs require a bona fide doctor-patient relationship, other common elements of clinical practice, such as those involving controlled substances, are much less common: only five states (Connecticut, Maryland, Minnesota, New Jersey, and New York) limit 30-day refills on marijuana access, and only three states (Connecticut, Massachusetts, and New York) require physicians to link to their state prescription drug monitoring program. Additionally, three states (Maryland, Massachusetts, and New York) require physician certification through a state-based licensing or training program. Finally, only two states (Minnesota and New York) require the provision of nonsmoked marijuana (such as cannabis-based edibles or tinctures). Many alternatives to smoking whole plant marijuana now exist—notably, vaporization with small portable devices—obviating the need for smoked marijuana (Hill 2015b; Kalant 2008).

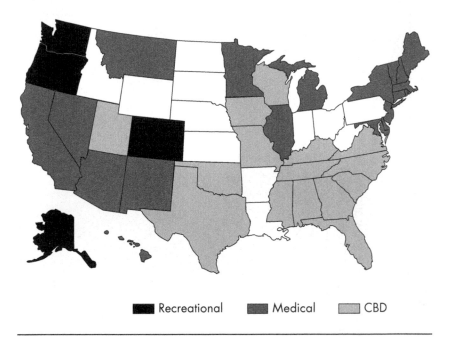

FIGURE 3–1. Marijuana laws by state, 2015.

All states with recreational marijuana laws also have medical marijuana laws. CBD=states with laws allowing for research with cannabidiol (CBD).

In sum, more than half of medical marijuana programs depart from a basic medical model; these states allow either home cultivation of marijuana or other forms of procurement outside of state-licensed manufacturing sites and do not include practices consistent with the basic standards of clinical care (Table 3–2). Among these medical marijuana programs, eight have established (optional) state-licensed dispensaries, and one (California) allows for dispensaries that are not regulated by the state (Bachhuber et al. 2014). Such "nonmedical" medical marijuana programs differ significantly with respect to route and year of passage from more medicalized programs (see Table 3–2). Specifically, medically oriented programs are more likely to have been passed by state legislatures than by voter initiatives (90% vs. 28.6%) and are more likely to have been passed in recent years.

There are 10 medically oriented medical marijuana programs—mostly passed since 2009—which typically require state-licensed production, manufacturing, dispensing, testing, and labeling of marijuana and derivative products. Half of these programs further include restrictive elements associated with controlled substances, such as linking to prescription drug monitoring programs or requiring physicians to complete specialized training courses.

TABLE 3–2. Medical marijuana program passage and characteristics

State (N=24)	Passage	State-licensed production required	Dispensaries allowed (*exclusive route of access)	Home grow allowed (*in locked facilities)	Limited to "30-day supply"	Registration fee ($)
Alaska	Voters (1998)			✓		25
Arizona	Voters (2010)		✓	✓*,a		75
California	Voters (1996)		✓	✓		33
Colorado	Voters (2000)		✓	✓		35
Connecticut	Legislature (2012)	✓	✓*		✓	100
Delaware	Legislature (2011)	✓	✓*			125
Hawaii	Legislature (2000)		✓	✓		25
Illinois	Legislature (2013)	✓	✓*			100
Maine	Voters (1999)		✓	✓*		
Maryland	Legislature (2014)	✓	✓*		✓	50

TABLE 3–2. Medical marijuana program passage and characteristics *(continued)*

State (*N*=24)	Passage	State-licensed production required	Dispensaries allowed (*exclusive route of access)	Home grow allowed (*in locked facilities)	Limited to "30-day supply"	Registration fee ($)
Massachusetts	Voters (2012)		✓	✓*,a		50
Michigan	Voters (2008)			✓*		25
Minnesota	Legislature (2014)	✓	✓*		✓	50
Montana	Voters (2004)		✓	✓		25
Nevada	Voters (2000)		✓	✓a		100
New Hampshire	Legislature (2013)	✓	✓*			TBD
New Jersey	Legislature (2010)	✓	✓*		✓	200
New Mexico	Legislature (2007)	✓	✓	✓a	✓	
New York	Legislature (2014)	✓	✓*		✓	50
Oregon	Voters (1998)		✓	✓b		20

TABLE 3–2. Medical marijuana program passage and characteristics (continued)

State (N=24)	Passage	State-licensed production required	Dispensaries allowed (*exclusive route of access)	Home grow allowed (*in locked facilities)	Limited to "30-day supply"	Registration fee ($)
Rhode Island	Legislature (2006)		✓	✓*		20
Vermont	Legislature (2004)		✓	✓*		50
Washington	Voters (1998)		✓	✓		
Washington, D.C.	Legislature (2010)	✓	✓*			25

Note. TBD=to be determined.

[a]Allowed only with a hardship exemption (i.e., living 25 miles from closest dispensary or financial hardship).

[b]Allowed only at registered grow sites, to produce for up to four people at a time.

Source. Data from the Marijuana Policy Project 2013, the National Conference of State Legislatures 2015, and ProCon.org 2015.

Such stark differences may be related to the process by which medical marijuana programs were established in each state. Early programs were mostly passed by voter initiatives in western states with low population density and depart from a medical model. Voter initiatives in many states (such as propositions in California) are typically difficult to scale back or regulate once passed (Caulkins et al. 2012b). More recent programs enacted by midwestern and northeastern state legislatures since 2009 are more highly regulated and more adherent to a medical model. These more recent programs typically require several years of work at the state level between initial passage and full implementation of a state-licensed manufacturing and dispensary system (in contrast to earlier programs, which simply permitted home cultivation or provided state-level legal protections for marijuana possession) (Pacula et al. 2014).

The effects of dispensaries on rates of marijuana use, heavy use, the use of high-potency strains, and associated changes in prices have received some attention in the medical and policy literature (Anderson and Rees 2014; Cerdá et al. 2012; Pacula et al. 2015). Epidemiological studies have been mixed in associating passage of medical marijuana laws with postimplementation changes in prevalence of use among adolescents and adults (Cerdá et al. 2012). One study found that dispensaries were associated with increased rates of heavy use of marijuana (Pacula et al. 2015). A second report, however, found no relationship between the implementation of dispensaries and rates of marijuana use (Anderson and Rees 2014).

Medical marijuana programs that establish dispensaries are mixed in their allowance of other means of marijuana procurement (see Table 3–2). For instance, many of the early medical marijuana programs established in states with higher rates of recreational marijuana use allowed home cultivation in addition to dispensaries (Sevigny et al. 2014). Such arrangements may confound the impact of dispensaries on access to marijuana. Although the presence of dispensaries may increase access (especially to high-potency marijuana products) or lower costs (and possibly concomitantly increase use or heavy use of marijuana), lower rates of program enrollment may result from state-licensed dispensaries when the latter are the exclusive route of access to medical marijuana. It may be that the mere presence of dispensaries has less influence on rates of use than eligibility requirements restricting who legitimately qualifies as a medical marijuana patient. If so, restrictions on access have direct implications for the role of physicians as gatekeepers (Appel 2008; Gambino 2013; Wilkinson and D'Souza 2014).

The cost of entry to medical marijuana programs is also significantly associated with enrollment rates, suggesting price sensitivity of demand for medical marijuana. States range in their fee schedules, with some charging nothing, and others, such as New Jersey, requiring a $200 fee from patients (although this fee can be reduced to $20 for those in specific state and federal assistance programs like the New Jersey Medicaid program) as part of registration (see Table 3–2). Registration fees, however, are unlikely to deter potential patients from enrollment given the relatively low price elasticity of demand for traditional medical treatments (compared with consumer goods or recreational drug use) (Caulkins et al. 2012a; Ringel et al. 2005).

Official rates of enrollment were notably low in all medical marijuana programs before 2009 (Anderson and Rees 2014), given the great uncertainty around the prospect of federal prosecution of medical marijuana programs and enrolled patients (Bachhuber et al. 2014). Following U.S. Department of Justice memos in 2009 and 2011, which provided uniform guidance to focus federal prosecutions and helped relieve states' concerns over possible investigations by clarifying federal intentions to refrain from interfering with lawfully run medical marijuana programs (Ogden 2009; Sznitman and Zolotov 2015), states operationalized dispensaries in greater numbers, facilitating consequent expansion of patient enrollment (Bachhuber et al. 2014; Pacula et al. 2015).

Indications. States have tended to include a common set of indications for participation in a medical marijuana program, including such diagnoses as cancer, HIV/AIDS, epilepsy, and amyotrophic lateral sclerosis accompanied by complications such as severe pain, nausea, and cachexia. Despite 20 years of medical marijuana programs, there remains limited high-quality evidence supporting the use of marijuana for many of the medical purposes for which participants seek program enrollment (Hill 2015b; Institute of Medicine 1999; Whiting et al. 2015). Although details of indications, formulations, efficacy, and adverse effects of medical marijuana will be presented in Chapter 4 ("Medical Marijuana: Indications, Formulations, Efficacy, and Adverse Effects"), indications are also discussed briefly here given the policy relevance.

To date, there is no evidence suggesting a psychiatric indication for medical marijuana use. Rather, several studies of moderate to high quality suggest that regular, and especially heavy, use of marijuana can cause and worsen affective, anxiety, and psychotic symptoms (Crippa et al. 2009; Degenhardt et al. 2003; Moore et al. 2007; Volkow et al. 2014). Nonetheless, posttraumatic stress disorder (PTSD) has been adopted by five states as an indication for qualification in a medical marijuana program (Bonn-Miller et al. 2014) (Table 3–3). Unfortunately, there is emerging concern that marijuana use can worsen PTSD (as with depression or anxiety) and that cannabis use disorder among patients with PTSD is much harder to treat (Boden et al. 2013). Additionally, patients with a comorbid mental illness such as a mood, anxiety, or substance use disorder are generally considered poor candidates for medical marijuana given the side-effect profile (Hill 2015a; Whiting et al. 2015).

TABLE 3–3.	Indications for medical marijuana program enrollment and associated levels of clinical evidence		
State	Indications with moderate- to high-quality evidence	Indications with limited evidence	Indications with little or no evidence
Alaska	Severe pain (cancer), spasticity (MS)	Severe nausea (HIV/AIDS), cachexia	Glaucoma, seizures
Arizona	Severe pain (cancer), spasticity (ALS)	Severe nausea (HIV/AIDS), cachexia	Alzheimer's disease, HCV
California	Severe pain (cancer), spasticity (MS)	Severe nausea (AIDS), cachexia, anorexia	Glaucoma, seizures, arthritis, migraine, "other chronic or persistent medical symptoms"
Colorado	Severe pain (cancer), spasticity (MS)	Severe nausea (AIDS), cachexia, anorexia	Glaucoma
Connecticut	Severe pain (cancer), spasticity (MS, spinal cord injury with objective evidence)	HIV/AIDS, cachexia	Glaucoma, seizures, Parkinson's disease, PTSD
Delaware	Severe pain[a] (cancer), spasticity (MS)	Severe nausea (HIV/AIDS), cachexia	Seizures, Alzheimer's disease, ALS, HCV
Hawaii	Severe pain (cancer), spasticity (MS)	Severe nausea (HIV/AIDS), cachexia	Glaucoma, seizures, Crohn's disease

TABLE 3–3. Indications for medical marijuana program enrollment and associated levels of clinical evidence *(continued)*

State	Indications with moderate- to high-quality evidence	Indications with limited evidence	Indications with little or no evidence
Illinois	Cancer, spasticity (MS, myoclonus, spinocerebellar ataxia, dystonia, muscular dystrophy, and spinal cord injury or disease), severe pain (including severe fibromyalgia and rheumatoid arthritis), neuropathic pain	HIV/AIDS, cachexia, Tourette syndrome	Glaucoma, ALS, Alzheimer's disease, HCV, Parkinson's disease, Tarlov cysts, hydromyelia/syringomyelia, fibrous dysplasia, TBI and postconcussion syndrome, Arnold-Chiari malformation and syringomyelia, neurofibromatosis, Sjögren's syndrome, lupus, interstitial cystitis, hydrocephalus, myasthenia gravis, nail-patella syndrome
Maine	Cancer, spasticity (MS)	Severe nausea (AIDS)	Glaucoma, seizures
Maryland	Severe pain, spasticity	Severe nausea, cachexia, anorexia	Seizures
Massachusetts	Cancer, spasticity (MS)	HIV/AIDS	Glaucoma, ALS, HCV, Parkinson's disease, Crohn's disease, "other conditions as determined in writing by a qualifying patient's physician"
Michigan	Severe pain (cancer), spasticity (MS)	Severe nausea (HIV/AIDS), cachexia	Glaucoma, seizures, HCV, Crohn's disease, Alzheimer's disease, PTSD, nail-patella syndrome
Minnesota	Severe pain (cancer), spasticity (MS)	HIV/AIDS, Tourette syndrome	Glaucoma, ALS, Crohn's disease, seizures, terminal illness with a life expectancy of <12 months

TABLE 3–3. Indications for medical marijuana program enrollment and associated levels of clinical evidence *(continued)*

State	Indications with moderate- to high-quality evidence	Indications with limited evidence	Indications with little or no evidence
Montana	Severe pain (cancer), spasticity (MS)	Severe nausea (HIV/AIDS), cachexia	Glaucoma, seizures, Crohn's disease
Nevada	Severe pain (cancer), spasticity	Severe nausea (AIDS), cachexia	Glaucoma, PTSD
New Hampshire	Severe pain[a] (cancer), spasticity (MS, muscular dystrophy, spinal cord injury or disease)	Severe nausea (HIV/AIDS), cachexia, anorexia	Glaucoma and elevated intraocular pressure, seizures, ALS, HCV, Crohn's disease, Alzheimer's disease, TBI, chronic pancreatitis
New Jersey	Severe pain (cancer), spasticity (MS, muscular dystrophy)	Severe nausea (HIV/AIDS), cachexia	Glaucoma, seizures, ALS, IBD, terminal illness (physician-determined prognosis of <12 months of life)
New Mexico	Severe pain (cancer), spasticity (MS, cervical dystonia, spinal cord injury), neuropathic pain	Severe nausea (HIV/AIDS), cachexia, anorexia	Glaucoma, seizures, ALS, HCV, Parkinson's disease, PTSD, Huntington's disease, inflammatory autoimmune-mediated arthritis, hospice care
New York	Cancer, spasticity (MS, spinal cord injury), neuropathic pain	HIV/AIDS	Seizures, ALS, Parkinson's disease, IBD, HCV, Huntington's disease; "The Department of Health commissioner…must decide whether to add Alzheimer's disease, muscular dystrophy, dystonia, PTSD, and rheumatoid arthritis within 18 months"
Oregon	Severe pain (cancer), spasticity (MS)	Severe nausea (HIV/AIDS), cachexia	Glaucoma, seizures

TABLE 3–3. Indications for medical marijuana program enrollment and associated levels of clinical evidence (continued)

State	Indications with moderate- to high-quality evidence	Indications with limited evidence	Indications with little or no evidence
Rhode Island	Severe pain (cancer), spasticity (MS)	Severe nausea (HIV/AIDS), cachexia	Glaucoma, seizures, HCV, Crohn's disease, Alzheimer's disease
Vermont	Severe pain (cancer), spasticity (MS)	Severe nausea (HIV/AIDS), cachexia	Seizures
Washington	Severe pain (cancer) (unrelieved by standard treatment), spasticity (MS)	Severe nausea (HIV/AIDS), cachexia, anorexia	Glaucoma, seizures, HCV, Crohn's disease, chronic renal failure
Washington, D.C.	Cancer, spasticity (MS)	Severe nausea (HIV/AIDS)	Glaucoma

Note. This table has been formatted to use consistent terminology to accurately reflect state policies but also allow for comparisons. Indications have been grouped according to level of evidence, given the current state of research, and are listed roughly in order of the frequency of inclusion across state programs. To better allow comparisons between states, some language was simplified; for instance, "spasticity" represents any indications pertaining to spasticity or persistent or intractable spasms. Often, states specify that a complication such as spasticity may be due to diagnoses such as multiple sclerosis (MS) or Crohn's disease. In these cases, the specific diagnoses included in the state's official list of conditions is mentioned by name parenthetically according to the existing level of evidence supporting their inclusion as an indication for medical marijuana. (For instance, there have been studies with positive findings for the treatment of spasticity due to MS but not spasticity due to Crohn's disease.) When diagnoses (such as Alzheimer's disease) were included for ambiguous reasons, they were listed in the table in the "little or no evidence" column unless there is a commonly associated complication with an evidence base (such as nausea related to advanced HIV/AIDS). ALS=amyotrophic lateral sclerosis; HCV=hepatitis C virus; IBD=inflammatory bowel disease; MS=multiple sclerosis; PTSD=posttraumatic stress disorder; TBI=traumatic brain injury.

[a]Severe pain that has not responded to previously prescribed medication or surgical measures, or for which other treatment options produced serious adverse effects.

Source. Data from Hill 2015b; Whiting et al. 2015.

Recent systematic reviews published in *JAMA* found that high-quality evidence for cannabinoids was limited to severe pain syndromes, neuropathic pain, and spasticity such as that due to multiple sclerosis (Hill 2015b; Whiting et al. 2015); the reviews did not include indications such as nausea and appetite stimulation for which FDA-approved medications are already on the market. These reviews, like many others, evaluated cannabinoids, including smoked medical marijuana, but were primarily evaluating trials with FDA-approved medications that are synthetic analogues to Δ^9-tetrahydrocannabinol (THC), such as dronabinol or nabilone (or nabiximols, a sublingual spray comprising THC and cannabidiol [CBD], which is not yet approved in the United States). The companion review and meta-analysis by Whiting and colleagues (2015) found moderate- to high-quality evidence for the use of cannabinoids for chronic pain and spasticity and low-quality evidence for nausea, cachexia, sleep disorders, and Tourette syndrome.

Table 3–3 lists the indications for medical marijuana by state. There is currently a disconnect between indications for medical marijuana with an evidence base and the qualifications for seeking enrollment in medical marijuana programs. Initial studies of program participants have shown that the typical medical marijuana patient is a young male with a nonspecific "chronic or severe pain" indication, without a formal diagnosis or prior trials of conventional treatments and with a history of recreational marijuana use, rather than an older adult with a terminal illness under intensive medical care (Bachhuber et al. 2014; Boden et al. 2013; Bonn-Miller et al. 2014; Reinarman et al. 2011). In fact, hundreds of thousands of medical marijuana program participants in states with looser regulations are thought to have been enrolled through medical marijuana specialty clinics staffed with their own physicians who certify patients for eligibility on the basis of patient self-report and outside clinic records (Crombie 2012).

A study by Walsh et al. (2013) found that among 600 Canadian users of marijuana in medical marijuana programs, it was difficult to differentiate characteristics of participants on the basis of authorized versus unauthorized use. In other words, the great majority of medical marijuana users had histories of recreational use, and the recreational users in the study endorsed comparable motivations for recreational marijuana use, such as help with pain, anxiety, and sleep, as did the medical marijuana program participants. A study from a Michigan dispensary found that 87% of patients were enrolled for "pain relief" and that many of the participants had concomitant use of opioids for pain (about half of whom also reported wanting to cut down on their use of prescription pain pills, suggesting that medical marijuana programs may be hot zones for identifying patients with difficulty controlling chronic opioid use) (Ilgen et al. 2013). Studies from the United Kingdom also indicate pain as the most common indication (Ware et al. 2005).

Reimbursement.   On the issue of who pays for medical marijuana and for which conditions, insurance reimbursement for medical marijuana has yet to arrive, and it is likely untenable given the current federal illegality of marijuana use in the United States (Pacula et al. 2014). Nonetheless, several jurisdictions have provisions in place explicitly protecting health insurers from liability for claims associated with medical marijuana. Practically speaking, even in jurisdictions where health insurers are explicitly free of liability, physicians cannot prescribe marijuana, and thus, there are no claims to send to the insurer.

Alternatives to insurance reimbursement exist. Some localities, such as the city of Berkeley in California and the state of Massachusetts, have passed compassionate access initiatives to provide lower-cost or free marijuana to low-income or impoverished patients (which inadvertently creates incentives to resell low-cost medical marijuana; see Hill 2015a). Additionally, 15 states allow for home cultivation of marijuana plants, which greatly reduces costs for participants who chose to home grow (4 of these states, however, allow home cultivation only when certain requirements, such as living more than 25 miles from a dispensary, are met; see Table 3–2).

Physician liability.   Despite the growing presence of medical marijuana programs across the country and the tremendous increase in participant enrollment since 2009, there remain uncertainties about the legal liability of physicians who recommend or certify patients for participation. After California first legalized medical marijuana in 1996, the federal government threatened to take away the medical licenses of physicians who recommended the use of marijuana (and raided some medical marijuana clinics). On October 29, 2002, a U.S. Court of Appeals (Ninth Circuit) ruling in the case *Conant v. Walters* restricted the federal government from "either revoking a physician's license to prescribe controlled substances or conducting an investigation of a physician that might lead to such revocation, where the basis for the government's action is solely the physician's professional 'recommendation' of the use of medical marijuana." The U.S. Supreme Court denied an appeal; therefore, physicians maintained the right to discuss marijuana with their patients. Nonetheless, the U.S. Drug Enforcement Administration (DEA) has been known, as recently as June 2014, to directly confront physicians who are working with medical marijuana dispensaries at their homes and offices (such as in Massachusetts) with ultimatums to either sever their ties to dispensaries or relinquish their DEA licenses (Lazar and Murphy 2014).

The legal implications of certifying patients (or certifying caregivers as is required of physicians in some states, such as Connecticut) for medical marijuana also remain unclear given the differences between the views of states versus the federal government. Marijuana is classified as a Schedule I substance, meaning that it has no currently accepted medical use and a high potential for abuse from a federal perspective. The prescription, supply, or sale of marijuana is illegal by federal law according to the Controlled Substances Act of 1970. Furthermore, it is not known to what extent, if any, a physician who certifies a patient for medical marijuana may be liable for negative outcomes (e.g., motor vehicle crashes or psychiatric adverse effects) (D'Souza and Ranganathan 2015). It is not known if malpractice insurance will cover liability attributable to physicians certifying medical marijuana use, and no case law yet exists to provide guidance.

Laws Pertaining to Cannabidiol

As of the time of this writing, 15 states have laws that recognize the therapeutic potential of high-potency CBD strains of marijuana (see Figure 3–1). In 2014, 11 states (Alabama, Florida, Iowa, Kentucky, Mississippi, Missouri, North Carolina, South Carolina, Tennessee, Utah, and Wisconsin) first enacted bills intended to allow at least some patients (such as those in university-sponsored clinical trials) to use isolated CBD products or high-CBD marijuana (Marijuana Policy Project 2014). The following year, 4 additional states (Georgia, Oklahoma, Texas, and Virginia) passed CBD-friendly laws. However, with the exception of Missouri and possibly Florida, these states do not include means for actually accessing marijuana. For instance, some of the programs limit access to physicians and pharmacies with an investigational drug (IND) permit from the FDA for a CBD-based product. Other programs restrict access to patients who purchase at an out-of-state medical marijuana dispensary that allows for out-of-state patients to both use their dispensaries and move marijuana across state borders (National Conference of State Legislatures 2015). Such stipulations are typically not allowable, and these CBD programs generally do not provide for an in-state marijuana production mechanism.

The Veterans Affairs Health Care System

Physicians working in the U.S. Department of Veterans Affairs (VA) health care system operate under different rules, given that the VA is federally managed. As a result, VA physicians have long been banned from recommending medical marijuana to patients who ask about it, even in states with legal programs. In 2014 and 2015, the U.S. House of Representatives narrowly defeated bills that would have effectively lifted the ban on VA physicians recommending marijuana to patients in the 23 states with medical marijuana programs. Although VA physicians cannot certify their patients, veterans now have the option of going outside of VA services and finding private physicians to help them gain access. However, it was not until 2010 that the VA released a statement that veterans who participate in legal state medical marijuana programs would no longer be disqualified from substance abuse and pain control programs through the VA.

Summary

The lack of data concerning medical marijuana programs involving roughly one million participants at the time of this writing (the great majority of whom are in non–medically oriented programs) and an unknown number of involved physicians is a strong argument for better and consistent state reporting on program activity and for longitudinal research. Many medical and professional societies have called for high-quality research into the potential therapeutic applications of marijuana. There is also a need for population-level research to assess the impact of medical marijuana programs once they are enacted.

Recreational Marijuana

With the legalization of marijuana for recreational use by adults over 21 years of age in four states and the District of Columbia as of November 2014, the United States entered a new era of drug control policy. There has been a slow, decades-long reversal of marijuana prohibition, with physicians enlisted as gatekeepers to legal access to marijuana for medical purposes, possibly as a precursor to recreational decriminalization and legalization.

Teasing Apart Decriminalization and Commercial Legalization

Since the first wave of decriminalization laws from the 1970s went into effect, a total of 20 states have, at the time of this writing, reduced penalties for first-time simple possession of marijuana (i.e., for personal consumption) to that of a traffic ticket, meaning no threat of felony convictions or prison time. (However, 5 of these states still classify possession as a criminal misdemeanor, although the offenses do not carry the risk of incarceration.) The enforcement of these laws varies. For instance, even though New York State had "decriminalized" marijuana possession for many years, it was common practice until recently for law enforcement to arrest individuals for marijuana possession during stop-and-frisk procedures.

Between 2012 and 2014, Colorado, Washington, Alaska, Oregon, and the District of Columbia went much further than decriminalization and voted to legalize adult use (over age 21) of recreational marijuana (see Figure 3–1). These five jurisdictions differ in their legislation and will likely experience different population-level effects of their reforms based on how they choose to approach regulations for production, sales, and advertising.

There are several models of legalization that do not a priori involve corporate commercialization (Reuter 2014). Primarily, there are two options that have not garnered much attention yet, which provide routes of legalization that may limit widespread increases in marijuana use by avoiding mass commercialization and marketing: 1) state monopoly systems and 2) "grow your own" policies that prohibit commercial sales but permit "gifting" of small amounts of marijuana (Reuter 2014).

Allowing for the sale of marijuana in commercial stores (vs. state-operated stores) will likely lead to much higher rates of use and possibly higher rates of heavy use as well. A recent example from alcohol control policy reform in Washington State gives insight. Costco was a major funder of a 2011 initiative to dismantle Washington State's requirement that liquor be sold through state-licensed stores. As a result, liquor sales increased despite higher privatized prices when the number of stores selling liquor in the state ballooned from 330 to 1,500 (Room 2014). (For alternatives to commercial sales, see Caulkins et al. 2012b for a more detailed discussion of home-grow and co-operative-gifting arrangements.)

It is hard to predict what these states will experience regarding changes in price for recreational marijuana. The expectation of legalization is that it may drop prices for marijuana 80%–90% because of decreased risk, increased automation, and economies of scale. The typical price elasticity of demand (percent change in consumption divided by percent change in price) for marijuana ranges between –0.002 and –0.7, depending on the population studied, with a narrower range of –0.3 to –0.5 for youth; these are roughly the same as the corresponding estimated ranges for cigarette price elasticity (Caulkins et al. 2012b). However, consumption of marijuana, like that of other drugs of abuse, is heavily concentrated among a minority of the heaviest users. As a result, the response of this group of users to changes in price most dominates how a price change will affect the overall quantity of marijuana consumed. For tobacco and alcohol, the elasticity of the total quantity consumed among heavy users is thought to be double that of the general population, meaning that these substances are more sensitive to small changes in price (Caulkins et al. 2012b). On the basis of the evidence available for marijuana, Pacula and Sevigny (2014) judged that the total price elasticity of demand around the current price of marijuana might be between –0.4 and –1.2.

Given the complexities of the intermingled finances of the emerging legal commercial market and persistent black market activity, it is unlikely that there is one pricing scheme or tax rate that simultaneously maximizes tax revenues and minimizes consumption given the inevitable rise in illicit activity that accompanies higher prices (as is seen currently with cigarette sales and illegal trafficking across state lines). A public health approach would ideally consider tax rates that also reflect THC potency or even the full cannabinoid profile of the product.

Colorado and Washington: Two Case Studies

Colorado citizens passed Constitutional Amendment 64 in November 2012 allowing for home cultivation of up to six marijuana plants and state-level control over the establishment of a retail recreational marijuana market overseen by the Colorado Department of Revenue, which also manages alcohol and tobacco licensing and enforcement (Room 2014). Recreational stores ("rec stores") were anticipated to open in approximately 20 cities and are prohibited from selling any additional merchandise; however, they can operate out of the same facility as a medical marijuana dispensary. No on-site consumption is allowed, and the quantity of marijuana eligible for purchase is one ounce for state residents and a quarter ounce for out-of-state tourists. Policies enhancing labeling of contents, ensuring childproof packaging, requiring warning labels, and clarifying taxes continue to evolve following high-profile deaths from marijuana-based edibles and complications following early recreational sales.

Contemporaneous with Colorado, Washington State passed a bill to allow for sales of marijuana for recreational use to be licensed by the state's Liquor Control Board without an allowance for home growing (Room 2014). Washington's approach mirrored much of the initial plan in Colorado but explicitly created a taxation scheme, as well as regulations on driving under the influence, restricting blood levels of THC to below 5 ng/mL. (However, studies to date have not shown a clear relationship between THC blood levels and functional impairment.) Rather than allowing counties to determine the number of rec stores, the Liquor Control Board maintains that authority and will allow for stores to operate until midnight, likely much later than in Colorado, as an attempt to better compete with the black market (Room 2014).

Following Colorado and Washington, voters in Alaska, Oregon, and the District of Columbia passed legalization in November 2014 (although the D.C. legislation is likely to be blocked by Congress for a period of time). These states are in the process of putting together a regulatory framework for implementing legalization.

International Perspectives

Conversations about drug control policies in the United States frequently reference international models. However, there is often confusion about what is actually allowable in other countries and how these regimes have evolved over time. The following three international examples highlight some of the decisions that states are facing when reforming marijuana laws and how different policies can affect the public.

United Kingdom. According to the Misuse of Drugs Act of 1971, controlled substances in the United Kingdom are classified into three classes (A, B, or C), which are similar to those in the scheduling system used in the United States regarding potential harmfulness. Following 4 years of protracted bureaucratic debate, in January 2004, British officials downgraded marijuana from Class B to C, prompting local news coverage to declare that marijuana was effectively decriminalized and leading to the resignation of Britain's top drug control governmental official in disagreement (Shiner 2015). Subsequently, new data emerged in the medical literature about the risk of psychosis and psychiatric side effects from marijuana use (Moore et al. 2007; Volkow et al. 2014), and the government in 2009 reclassified marijuana as Class B.

The Netherlands. Since 1976, the Netherlands has chosen not to enforce laws pertaining to marijuana, leading to a de facto legalization of adult possession and use (Nordstrom and Kleber 2011; Pardo 2014). Technically, under Dutch law, the wholesale cultivation, processing, and "backdoor" sale of marijuana to retail outlets remains illegal, and the law is intermittently enforced, keeping prices high (Pardo 2014; Transform Drug Policy Foundation 2009). Under this system, commercial advertising began to expand, and marijuana use among Dutch youth increased by 200% between 1984 and 1992 (whereas use decreased by 66% during this time in the United States) (Nordstrom and Kleber 2011). As a result, in 1996 the Dutch Parliament attempted to close half of the operating coffeeshops where marijuana is available for purchase, with only limited success (only 10% eventually closed) and reduce the amount of marijuana customers could buy.

The Dutch experience suggests that once mass marketing is allowed, it will affect rates of use, and therefore, once a substance is legalized, commercial interests can greatly influence attempts to rein in activity (Nordstrom and Kleber 2011). Currently, coffeeshops in the Netherlands are banned from advertising in mass media. This restriction was intended to especially limit use among youth; however, such a ban would not necessarily hold up to judicial scrutiny in the United States, which has a track record of aggressively protecting corporations' rights to free speech (Caulkins et al. 2012b). Additional restrictions have been added to the Dutch system in recent years, such as requiring proof of residence, but these policies are inconsistently enforced (Hill 2015a).

Uruguay. Uruguay is the first and only nation to attempt to regulate the entire marijuana market for nonmedical purposes since ratification of the

United Nations Single Convention on Narcotic Drugs of 1961 (Pardo 2014). Unlike the trend among reform-minded states in the United States, Uruguay's initiative was developed in 2012 by the executive branch in conjunction with the legislature rather than by voter referendum (Pardo 2014). The system authorized under outgoing president José Mujica (2010–2015) intended to allow three options of procurement for citizens or legal residents: 1) home grow (up to six plants), 2) cooperatives with up to 45 members, and 3) licensed production facilities that must sell wholesale directly to the government (Room 2014). A newly created government institute, the Institute of Regulation and Control of Cannabis, oversees sales through pharmacies and limits dispensing to a maximum of 40 g (about 1.5 ounces) to consumers who have registered with a confidential state-run registry (Room 2014). The government plans to prohibit any promotion or advertising and will likely impose taxes, but developments have stalled because of the new president's resistance to recreational sales through state-licensed pharmacies. As of spring 2015, only the home-grow option has been fully implemented for residents who request a permit from the Institute of Regulation at a local post office. Cooperatives face bureaucratic hurdles, and concerns have emerged that a gray market will appear for local citizens capitalizing on a chance to resell marijuana to tourists.

Summary

Although there is much to learn about drug control policy and the nuances of marijuana policy reform across different sociocultural settings, there remain many more questions than answers when it comes to the myriad changes rapidly occurring across the United States and their potential impact on patients, families, and providers.

Synthetic Cannabinoids: New Threats

Synthetic cannabinoids are discussed in detail in Chapter 7 ("Synthetic Cannabinoids: Emergence, Epidemiology, and Clinical Effects and Management"). Federal and state authorities are now in a constant race to identify and outlaw new synthetic and "designer" drugs. Synthetic cannabinoids in particular have become popular throughout the United States, especially in low-income communities. The Synthetic Drug Abuse Prevention Act was part of the FDA Safety and Innovation Act of 2012 and permanently placed 26 types of synthetic cannabinoids (and cathinones, colloquially known as "bath salts") into Schedule I. In each of the following 2 years, the DEA used emergency scheduling and other authority to classify additional synthetic cannabinoids as Schedule I controlled substances. However, even after novel substances are molecularly identified, new emergency laws attempting to ban them are difficult to enforce.

Conclusion

There are several important points of which the physician treating Marcus from the opening clinical vignette should be aware. Although physicians do not have legal authority to prescribe medical marijuana anywhere in the United States, 23 states and the District of Columbia permit, at the time of this writing, physicians to "recommend" marijuana to patients with a qualifying condition. However, the states are inconsistent in the indications they include as qualifying, and there is little relationship between what is allowable under state law and the current evidence base. To date, there are no psychiatric indications for medical marijuana, and there is a growing literature indicating that heavy or prolonged marijuana use can worsen symptoms of psychotic, anxiety, mood, trauma-related, and substance use disorders. Patients with a history of substance use disorders in particular are poor candidates for being treated with a substance that has uncertain benefits and clinically significant psychiatric side effects and abuse liability. Furthermore, the liability to physicians who recommend medical marijuana is unknown and may change as state and federal policies evolve.

Although four states and the District of Columbia have legalized the adult use of recreational marijuana, no states currently allow individuals to transport marijuana across state lines. States that now allow both medical marijuana and recreational sales are struggling with models of production, sales, and taxation that minimize risks to the public while also containing black market activity. Although there are some lessons to be gleaned from other countries such as the United Kingdom, the Netherlands, and Uruguay, the United States is now a world leader in reforming marijuana control laws. As states' policies continue to evolve, much will be learned about the true demand curve for both medical and recreational marijuana.

Key Points

- In the mid-twentieth century, the United States led the world in marijuana prohibition and promoted the United Nations Single Convention on Narcotic Drugs, but the country is now experiencing a wave of new policies and approaches to legalizing both medical and recreational marijuana use at the state level.

- Despite 20 years of medical marijuana programs, there is minimal evidence for many indications allowed under state law, and physician liability remains uncertain.
- Currently, there is no psychiatric indication for medical marijuana; however, five states include posttraumatic stress disorder (PTSD) as a qualifying condition for program enrollment, despite evidence that marijuana may worsen the course of illness for patients with psychiatric conditions such as PTSD, depression, anxiety, and psychosis.
- There is no standard model for legalization, and currently, each state legalizing recreational use of marijuana among adults is designing its own approach. However, there is broad anticipation of price reductions, a likely decrease in perceptions of harm, an increase in high-potency marijuana strains, and resultant increased rates of use and heavy use among the public.

References

Anderson DM, Rees DI: Medical marijuana laws, traffic fatalities, and alcohol consumption. Discussion Paper Series IZA DP No 6112. Bonn, Germany, Institute for the Study of Labor, 2011. Available at: http://ftp.iza.org/dp6112.pdf. Accessed November 21, 2015.

Anderson DM, Rees DI: The role of dispensaries: the devil is in the details. J Policy Anal Manage 33(1):235–240, 2014 24358532

Appel J: Physicians are not bootleggers. Bull Hist Med 82(2):355–386, 2008 18622072

Bachhuber MA, Saloner B, Cunningham CO, et al: Medical cannabis laws and opioid analgesic overdose mortality in the United States, 1999–2010. JAMA Intern Med 174(10):1668–1673, 2014 25154332

Barcott B: Weed the People: The Future of Legal Marijuana in America. New York, Time, 2015

Baum D: Smoke and Mirrors: The War on Drugs and the Politics of Failure. New York, Back Bay Books, 1997

Boden MT, Babson KA, Vujanovic AA, et al: Posttraumatic stress disorder and cannabis use characteristics among military veterans with cannabis dependence. Am J Addict 22(3):277–284, 2013 23617872

Bonn-Miller MO, Boden MT, Bucossi MM, et al: Self-reported cannabis use characteristics, patterns and helpfulness among medical cannabis users. Am J Drug Alcohol Abuse 40(1):23–30, 2014 24205805

Caulkins JP, Hawken A, Kilmer B, et al: Marijuana Legalization: What Everyone Needs to Know. New York, Oxford University Press, 2012a

Caulkins JP, Kilmer B, MacCoun RJ, et al: Design considerations for legalizing cannabis: lessons inspired by analysis of California's Proposition 19. Addiction 107(5):865–871, 2012b 21985069

Cerdá M, Wall M, Keyes KM, et al: Medical marijuana laws in 50 states: investigating the relationship between state legalization of medical marijuana and marijuana use, abuse and dependence. Drug Alcohol Depend 120(1–3):22–27, 2012 22099393

Choi A: The impact of medical marijuana laws on marijuana use and other risky health behaviors. Doctoral dissertation, Department of Policy Analysis and Management, Cornell University, 2014

Courtwright D: Forces of Habit: Drugs and the Making of the Modern World. Boston, MA, Harvard University Press, 2002

Crippa JA, Zuardi AW, Martín-Santos R, et al: Cannabis and anxiety: a critical review of the evidence. Hum Psychopharmacol 24(7):515–523, 2009 19693792

Crombie N: Medical marijuana: a few high-volume doctors approve most patients. The Oregonian/Oregon Live, December 29, 2012

Degenhardt L, Hall W, Lynskey M: Exploring the association between cannabis use and depression. Addiction 98(11):1493–1504, 2003 14616175

D'Souza DC, Ranganathan M: Medical marijuana: is the cart before the horse? JAMA 313(24):2431–2432, 2015 26103026

Federal Bureau of Investigation: Crime in the United States, 2001: FBI Uniform Crime Report. Washington, DC, U.S. Government Printing Office, 2001

Gambino M: During prohibition, your doctor could write you a prescription for booze. Smithsonian, October 7, 2013. Available at: http://www.smithsonian-mag.com/history/during-prohibition-your-doctor-could-write-you-prescription-booze-180947940/?no-ist. Accessed April 15, 2015.

Hill KP: Marijuana: The Unbiased Truth About the World's Most Popular Weed. Center City, MN, Hazelden, 2015a

Hill KP: Medical marijuana for treatment of chronic pain and other medical and psychiatric problems: a clinical review. JAMA 313(24):2474–2483, 2015b 26103031

Ilgen MA, Bohnert K, Kleinberg F, et al: Characteristics of adults seeking medical marijuana certification. Drug Alcohol Depend 132(3):654–659, 2013 23683791

Institute of Medicine: Marijuana and Medicine: Assessing the Science. Edited by Joy JE, Watson SJ Jr, Benson JA Jr. Washington, DC, National Academies Press, 1999

Kalant H: Smoked marijuana as medicine: not much future. Clin Pharmacol Ther 83(4):517–519, 2008 18349871

Lazar K, Murphy S: DEA targets doctors linked to medical marijuana. The Boston Globe, June 6, 2014

Marijuana Policy Project: State Medical Marijuana Programs' Financial Information. Washington, DC, Marijuana Policy Project, October 18, 2013. Available at http://www.mpp.org/issues/medical-marijuana/state-medical-marijuana-programs-financial-information/. Accessed April 15, 2015.

Marijuana Policy Project: Medical Dispensary Laws: Fees and Taxes, October 18, 2013. Washington, DC, Marijuana Policy Project, 2014. Available at: http://www.mpp.org/issues/medical-marijuana/. Accessed April 15, 2015.

Moore TH, Zammit S, Lingford-Hughes A, et al: Cannabis use and risk of psychotic or affective mental health outcomes: a systematic review. Lancet 370(9584):319–328, 2007 17662880

Musto DF: The American Disease: Origins of Narcotic Control. New York, Oxford
  University Press, 1999
National Commission on Marihuana and Drug Abuse: Marihuana: A Signal of Mis-
  understanding. U.S. Government Printing Office, Washington, DC, March 1972
National Conference of State Legislatures: State Medical Marijuana Laws. Washing-
  ton, DC, National Conference of State Legislatures, June 6, 2015. Available at:
  http://www.ncsl.org/research/health/state-medical-marijuana-laws.aspx. Ac-
  cessed November 21, 2015.
Nordstrom BR, Kleber HD: Clinical and societal implications of drug legalization, in
  Lowinson and Ruiz's Substance Abuse: A Comprehensive Textbook. Edited by
  Ruiz P, Strain E. New York, Lippincott Williams & Wilkins, 2011, pp 1032–1043
Ogden DW: Memorandum for Selected United States Attorneys: Investigations and
  Prosecutions in States Authorizing the Medical Use of Marijuana. U.S. Depart-
  ment of Justice Web site, October 19, 2009. Available at http://www.justice.gov/
  opa/blog/memorandum-selected-united-state-attorneys-investigations-and-
  prosecutions-states. Accessed January 7, 2016.
Pacula RL, Sevigny EL: Marijuana liberalization policies: why we can't learn much from
  policy still in motion. J Policy Anal Manage 33(1):212–221, 2014 24358530
Pacula RL, Hunt P, Boustead A: Words can be deceiving: a review of variation among
  legally effective medical marijuana laws in the United States. J Drug Policy Anal
  7(1):1–19, 2014 25657828
Pacula RL, Powell D, Heaton P, et al: Assessing the effects of medical marijuana laws
  on marijuana use: the devil is in the details. J Policy Anal Manage 34(1):7–31,
  2015 25558490
Pardo B: Cannabis policy reforms in the Americas: a comparative analysis of Colorado,
  Washington, and Uruguay. Int J Drug Policy 25(4):727–735, 2014 24970383
ProCon.org: Number of Legal Medical Marijuana Patients, October 27, 2014. Available
  at: http://medicalmarijuana.procon.org/view.resource.php?resourceID=005889.
  Accessed April 15, 2015.
Reinarman C, Nunberg H, Lanthier F, et al: Who are medical marijuana patients?
  Population characteristics from nine California assessment clinics. J Psychoac-
  tive Drugs 43(2):128–135, 2011 21858958
Reuter P: The difficulty of restricting promotion of legalized marijuana in the United
  States. Addiction 109(3):353–354, 2014 24524313
Ringel JS, Hosek SD, Vollaard BA, et al: The Elasticity of Demand for Health Care: A
  Review of the Literature and Its Application to the Military Health System. Santa
  Monica, CA, National Defense Research Institute, RAND, 2005
Room R: Legalizing a market for cannabis for pleasure: Colorado, Washington, Uru-
  guay and beyond. Addiction 109(3):345–351, 2014 24180513
Sevigny EL, Pacula RL, Heaton P: The effects of medical marijuana laws on potency.
  Int J Drug Policy 25(2):308–319, 2014 24502887
Shiner M: Drug policy reform and the reclassification of cannabis in England and
  Wales: a cautionary tale. Int J Drug Policy 26(7):696–704, 2015 25959525

Song A: How difficult is it to get a medical marijuana card? KATU News, May 20, 2010. Available at: http://katu.com/archive/how-difficult-is-it-to-get-a-medical-marijuana-card-11-19-2015. Accessed January 7, 2016.

Strang J, Babor T, Caulkins J, et al: Drug policy and the public good: evidence for effective interventions. Lancet 379(9810):71–83, 2012 22225672

Sznitman SR, Zolotov Y: Cannabis for therapeutic purposes and public health and safety: a systematic and critical review. Int J Drug Policy 26(1):20–29, 2015 25304050

Transform Drug Policy Foundation: After the War on Drugs: Blueprint for Regulation. Bristol, UK, Transform Drug Policy Foundation, 2009

Volkow ND, Baler RD, Compton WM, et al: Adverse health effects of marijuana use. N Engl J Med 370(23):2219–2227, 2014 24897085

Walsh Z, Callaway R, Belle-Isle L, et al: Cannabis for therapeutic purposes: patient characteristics, access, and reasons for use. Int J Drug Policy 24(6):511–516, 2013 24095000

Ware MA, Adams H, Guy GW: The medicinal use of cannabis in the UK: results of a nationwide survey. Int J Clin Pract 59(3):291–295, 2005

Whiting PF, Wolff RF, Deshpande S, et al: Cannabinoids for medical use: a systematic review and meta-analysis. JAMA 313(24):2456–2473, 2015 26103030

Wilkinson ST, D'Souza DC: Problems with the medicalization of marijuana. JAMA 311(23):2377–2378, 2014 24845238

CHAPTER 4

Medical Marijuana

Indications, Formulations, Efficacy, and Adverse Effects

Thida Thant, M.D.

Elin C. Kondrad, M.D.

Abraham M. Nussbaum, M.D., M.T.S.

Clinical Vignette: Jacob and a Request for Medical Marijuana

Dr. Tori Francis is an outpatient psychiatrist at a community mental health center. Her next patient, Jacob Darcy, is presenting for an intake visit. Jacob is a 30-year-old man with a history of bipolar disorder, generalized anxiety disorder, insomnia, and chronic back pain who moved to town 4 months ago. Since his arrival, he has struggled to secure employment and has experienced worsening anxiety and insomnia. In an effort to ameliorate his symptoms, he has increased his chronic marijuana use and is now using marijuana about three times daily.

On examination, Jacob appears casually dressed and appropriately groomed. He is cooperative, but his eye contact is intermittent. He demonstrates neither psychomotor agitation nor retardation. His speech is mildly increased in rate but is nonpressured and appropriate in volume. He describes his mood as "down," and he appears dysphoric in affect. His thought process is linear and goal directed. He denies suicidal or homicidal ideation, and he describes no perceptual disturbances or delusional thought content. His insight and judgment are fair.

As Dr. Francis performs the intake interview, she explores Jacob's psychiatric history. In college, Jacob exhibited an irritable, labile mood, and the phy-

71

sician at his school's student health center diagnosed him with bipolar disorder. However, Jacob denies discrete episodes of mania or hypomania and has never been hospitalized. Instead, he has received care from a series of primary care physicians who have diagnosed him with anxiety and insomnia and prescribed various antidepressants, along with trials of benzodiazepines and lithium. He did not find any of these medications helpful and discontinued most of them after a few weeks. In contrast, he has an extended history of marijuana use, beginning at age 15, and he says that marijuana manages his anxiety and mood symptoms. At present, he most commonly smokes joints (hand-rolled marijuana cigarettes), consumes edibles (food items infused or prepared with marijuana), or dabs (Δ^9-tetrahydrocannabinol [THC]-concentrated forms of marijuana extracted using solvents such as butane). He has experimented with other substances but does not use them consistently. His family psychiatric history is notable for anxiety on both his paternal and maternal sides. Some family members have benefited from psychotropic medications, but Jacob prefers marijuana as a "natural" medication. With direct questioning, he admits that despite his preference for marijuana, his anxiety and insomnia have increased as he has recently escalated his marijuana use. He wonders if Dr. Francis could recommend an alternative strain and formulation of marijuana and if Dr. Francis can help him get a medical marijuana card. He has tired of purchasing marijuana illicitly, but several of his friends use medical marijuana to alleviate a variety of medical issues, ranging from pain to nausea.

In places where medical marijuana is permitted, clinical presentations like Jacob's are increasingly common. Patients with psychiatric histories that are simultaneously lengthy and poorly characterized often present with reports of using marijuana for both medical and social reasons. In this case, Jacob reports 15 years of marijuana use, during which time he has accumulated multiple psychiatric diagnoses. In addition to performing a standard assessment for psychiatric and substance use disorders, health care practitioners are faced with a host of additional concerns when they evaluate such patients, including the following: What are the relationships between marijuana and mental illnesses? What are the medical and psychiatric indications for medical marijuana? What are the available formulations of medical marijuana, and what are their adverse effects?

Although most mental health professionals are comfortable assessing marijuana use, they are less informed regarding the medical marijuana literature and its answers to the aforementioned questions. In this chapter we guide practitioners through these questions using the most current literature available. Wherever possible, peer-reviewed literature is reported. In areas where there is no published peer-reviewed literature, we have drawn on non-peer-reviewed literature, where much of the current knowledge about medical marijuana formulations and use exists.

Cannabinoid Basics
and Formulations of Marijuana

The Basics of Cannabinoids

The human body's endogenous cannabinoid system and the receptors that bind both endogenous cannabinoids and the exogenous compounds in marijuana have been elucidated over the past quarter century. We know that marijuana contains hundreds of compounds, including many flavonoids and terpenoids, along with more than 70 known cannabinoids that affect the endocannabinoid system. The best-known cannabinoids are THC, which is responsible for many of marijuana's psychoactive properties, and cannabidiol (CBD), which is thought to have anti-inflammatory and anti-epileptic properties without the psychoactive and euphoric effects of THC. Other notable cannabinoids include Δ^8-tetrahydrocannabinol, cannabinol, cannabichromene, cannabigerol, cannabinodiol, and tetrahydrocannabivarin, although their effects on humans remain poorly elucidated (Burns and Ineck 2006). The ratio of THC to other cannabinoids varies between *Cannabis sativa* plant strains. Many growers and users of medical marijuana refer to these ratios, particularly the ratio of THC to CBD, when choosing between different strains of marijuana.

Pharmaceutical Formulations of Marijuana

Pharmaceutical companies have purified, tested, and marketed several cannabinoid formulations for human use, as detailed in Table 4–1. In the United States, two U.S. Food and Drug Administration (FDA)–approved drugs are currently available: dronabinol (Marinol) and nabilone (Cesamet), both U.S. Drug Enforcement Agency (DEA) Schedule II substances (i.e., deemed by the DEA to have a high potential for abuse but accepted for restricted medical use). Nabiximols (Sativex), although not available in the United States, is approved for use in 15 countries, including Canada and the United Kingdom. Cannabidiol (Epidiolex) is in Phase III investigational trials.

Dispensary Formulations of Marijuana

Purified and approved pharmaceuticals represent a small minority of the cannabinoids being used for medical purposes; most medical marijuana patients are smoking or otherwise consuming marijuana plant flowers and other nonpurified plant extracts. Because marijuana is still illegal at the federal level in the United States and in many other countries around the world,

TABLE 4–1.   Pharmaceutical formulations of cannabinoids

Product and chemical components	Indications	Dosing	Common side effects (experienced by >5% of patients)	Formulations and average wholesale price in the United States
Dronabinol (Marinol) Dronabinol (generic) *Synthetic THC*	AIDS-associated anorexia/ weight loss Chemotherapy-related nausea and vomiting	2.5–10 mg po bid 5 mg/m² po 1–3 hours before chemotherapy and every 2–4 hours after chemotherapy; up to 6 doses/day	Dizziness, somnolence, euphoria, paranoia, abdominal pain, weakness, nausea/ vomiting, tachycardia, anxiety, ataxia, confusion	2.5 mg generic capsule: $353.57 for 60 5 mg generic capsule: $735.85 for 60 10 mg generic capsule: $1,351.30 for 60
Nabilone (Cesamet) *Dibenzo(b,d)pyrans (synthetic cannabinoid chemically similar to THC)*	Chemotherapy-related nausea and vomiting	1–2 mg po bid; first dose 1–3 hours before chemotherapy	Drowsiness, dizziness, vertigo, euphoria, xerostomia, depression, ataxia, visual disturbance, impaired concentration, sleep disturbance, dysphoria, hypotension, weakness, anorexia, headache	1 mg tablet: $2,010.77 for 50

TABLE 4–1.   Pharmaceutical formulations of cannabinoids (*continued*)

Product and chemical components	Indications	Dosing	Common side effects (experienced by >5% of patients)	Formulations and average wholesale price in the United States
Nabiximols (Sativex)[a] *Purified marijuana plant extract; 1:1 ratio of cannabidiol:THC*	Refractory muscle spasticity in multiple sclerosis	2.5 mg cannabidiol and 2.7 mg THC per spray; up to 12 sprays per day	Dizziness, somnolence, fatigue, nausea, hypotension, confusion, vertigo, vomiting, diarrhea, xerostomia, urinary retention, abnormal liver function tests, weakness	Oromucosal spray
Cannabidiol (Epidiolex)[b] *Purified marijuana plant extract*	Refractory epilepsy, particularly in children with Dravet syndrome or Lennox-Gastaut syndrome	Undetermined	Undetermined	Liquid formulation

Note.   bid=twice a day; po=by mouth; THC=Δ^9-tetrahydrocannabinol.
[a]Not approved for use in the United States.
[b]Investigational agent, not yet approved in any country.
Source.   Lexicomp Online, http//online.lexi.com. Accessed June 22, 2015.

few medical practitioners are educated about the medical use of marijuana, and there are limited high-quality data available in the medical literature. However, in the countries and U.S. states that permit medical marijuana, marijuana shops (dispensaries) are ubiquitous. Because a remarkable array of formulations are available for purchase and consumption at these facilities, it is important for a practitioner to have a basic understanding of what cannabinoids patients can access.

Marijuana Strains and Varieties

There are hundreds of cultivated varieties of marijuana that are known by marijuana growers and users by names that describe their effects, such as Purple Haze, or their flavor, such as Sour Diesel. It remains unclear what biochemical differences exist between different cultivated varieties, so it is currently difficult to reliably describe medical differences, but growers and users report significant differences between varieties.

Growers and users often classify marijuana strains first on the basis of plant morphology; *Cannabis sativa* plants are taller with longer, thinner leaves than *Cannabis indica* plants. Although these morphological differences are not consistently associated with biochemical differences, growers and users describe *sativa*-dominant strains as characterized by a stimulating and energizing feeling and as more likely to induce hallucinogenic states. Because of these effects, many users prefer daytime use of *sativa* strains. *Sativa*-dominant strains typically have high THC:CBD ratios, and some users prefer using *sativa* strains to induce euphoria and a sense of well-being. *Indica*-dominant strains typically have comparatively lower THC:CBD ratios, and users often report that use of *indica* strains induces feelings of calm, relaxation, and sedation. They are sometimes used as an analgesic or a sleep aid (Pearce et al. 2014).

Additional Formulations

Although many people think of smoking as the primary way to use marijuana, there are many methods of ingesting or otherwise administering marijuana products. These can include smoked forms such as kief and hashish, topical forms using marijuana-infused oils, edible forms using food products infused with marijuana, and spray and sublingual forms using tinctures. These forms and their methods of administration are outlined in more detail in Table 4–2.

TABLE 4–2.   Medical marijuana formulations

	Description	Method of administration
Kief	Powder extracted from cannabinoid-rich glands of the cannabis plant (trichomes)	The powder can be smoked or compressed into cakes of hashish
Hashish	Concentrated trichomes with a higher THC content than plant material	Hashish is often smoked (using a vaporizer or hookah or in a joint) or mixed with food
Hash oil	A mix of essential oils and resins extracted from marijuana plants using solvents such as ethanol or butane	The solvent is evaporated, yielding an oil with a high concentration of THC that can be smoked with a special pipe (sometimes referred to as "dabbing"), vaporized, or infused into food
Edibles	Food products infused with marijuana	The food products may have marijuana added directly to them, or they may be made with butter, oil, or alcohol that has been infused with marijuana
Tincture	Cannabinoids extracted using alcohol	Tincture is used in liquid form and is absorbed through the mucous membranes of the mouth; it can also be administered sublingually in a spray form
Topicals	Salve or cream that can be applied topically	Topicals are usually made with an oil that is infused with marijuana

Note.   THC=Δ^9-tetrahydrocannabinol.
Source.   Americans for Safe Access 2015.

Metabolism and Monitoring

Pharmacokinetics

The pharmacokinetics of marijuana vary with route of administration. Because much of the THC content in smoked marijuana is dissipated in the smoke, the estimated bioavailability of smoked THC is 10%–25% (Borgelt et al. 2013). Inhaled marijuana reaches peak concentrations 3–10 minutes after smoking. Euphoric effects peak after 20–30 minutes and decline to low levels 3 hours after smoking (Grotenhermen 2003).

Orally ingested THC has a bioavailability of 5%–20% because of gastric degradation and extensive first-pass metabolism by the liver. Bioavailability is highly variable from one individual to another, which results in inconsistency in titration of edible marijuana products. The peak concentration of oral THC is delayed compared with inhaled THC and is reached in 1–3 hours. Psychotropic effects set in between 30 and 90 minutes, peak at 2–4 hours, and decline to low levels after approximately 6 hours (Grotenhermen 2003). The pharmacokinetics of different THC formulations are compared in Table 4–3. Like THC, CBD is lipophilic and has an oral bioavailability ranging from 13% to 19% (Borgelt et al. 2013).

Quality Control

Pharmaceutical forms of marijuana (e.g., dronabinol, nabilone) are standardized in formulation, composition, and dose in order to meet regulatory requirements for prescribing. The regulation of medical marijuana production, however, is both less stringent and more varied. Some of this variability derives from the difficulty of standardizing plant material, because the potency of marijuana is different between individual plants and even in different parts within the same plant. In the popular press (e.g., Baca 2015), there are credible reports of profound discrepancies between the potency claimed on product labels and the potency demonstrated in laboratory analyses of commercially available marijuana products. There is ample evidence that, through the efforts of marijuana breeders and growers, the potency of marijuana has increased substantially over the past 20 years, with an average THC content of less than 4% in 1995 compared with greater than 12% in 2012 (Volkow et al. 2014).

Because medical marijuana products are derived from plant material, they are also susceptible to contamination from pesticides, molds, fungi, and bacteria. Small studies have documented widespread *Aspergillus* contamination in particular, with evidence of contamination from this fungus in the majority of tested plant specimens and corresponding high levels of *Asper-*

TABLE 4–3. **Basic pharmacokinetics of smoked and orally ingested marijuana**

Route	Dose	Percent dose in plasma	Onset of pharmacologic action	Peak plasma levels
Smoked	13 mg	8%–24%	10 minutes	3 minutes
Oral (baked into cookies)	20 mg	4%–12%	120–180 minutes	60–120 minutes

Source. Ohlsson et al. 1980.

gillus antibodies found in marijuana users (McLaren et al. 2008). In the United States, there are no federal guidelines for the testing of medical marijuana for either potency or contaminants, and few state regulations exist. For example, Colorado has state-licensed testing facilities and requires testing of recreational marijuana products for potency, homogeneity, and contaminants (Brohl et al. 2015), but such regulations do not exist for the testing of medical marijuana products even though Colorado is considered to have the most regulated medical marijuana system in the United States. There are private laboratories that offer testing services, but the onus is presently on the growers or manufacturers to voluntarily pursue testing of their products.

Monitoring of Marijuana Use in the Clinical Setting

A practical concern for medical providers is the role of drug testing, and the interpretation of this testing, when it comes to evaluation of marijuana use. The most common and easily obtained drug test is the urine test that detects the nonpsychoactive marijuana metabolite THC carboxylic acid (THC-COOH). The length of time marijuana can be detected in the urine varies widely depending on frequency and duration of use. Because marijuana is lipophilic and is stored in body fat, chronic heavy users have been found to have positive urine drug screens up to 67 days after their last marijuana intake. In contrast, a naïve user may have a negative urine drug screen only hours after smoking marijuana (Huestis 2007). Therefore, a positive urine drug test for marijuana indicates that an individual has used marijuana, but it is not helpful in determining when the individual's last marijuana use was. It should be noted that in infrequent marijuana users, drug metabolites can take 1–4 hours to reach levels detectable by most urine drug tests (Huestis 2007). The Substance Abuse and Mental Health Services Administration recommends a cutoff concentration of 50 ng/mL for a positive result in a urine immunoassay test.

There are a variety of substances that can cause false positives in urine drug testing for marijuana, the most common of which are efavirenz (used in the treatment of HIV/AIDS) and proton pump inhibitors used to treat acid reflux and peptic ulcers, such as lansoprazole and omeprazole. Furthermore, the use of pharmaceutical formulations of marijuana (e.g., dronabinol, marketed as Marinol; nabilone, marketed as Cesamet) will result in a positive urine drug screen for marijuana and cannot be distinguished from the use of smoked or ingested marijuana in such testing. Sodium chloride, sodium hypochlorite, and liquid dishwashing detergent have all been found to reduce levels of detection of cannabinoids in urine drug screening when they are added to urine samples (Phan et al. 2012).

Blood testing for marijuana is more clearly correlated with time of use and level of impairment. THC levels peak quickly after a person smokes marijuana and are detectable for several hours in naïve users and up to 13 days in chronic heavy users. THC-COOH blood levels remain high for much longer than do THC levels, and mathematical models to determine time of last use have been developed using both THC levels alone and THC-COOH:THC ratios. THC blood levels in chronic users remain elevated for longer periods of time than those of naïve users but are often less than 2 ng/mL. THC-COOH levels remain significantly elevated for long periods of time in chronic users (Huestis 2007). A recent review of the effects of marijuana on driving skills suggested that a blood THC concentration of 2–5 ng/mL was correlated with significant driving impairment (Hartman and Huestis 2013).

Testing of saliva, which has the clear advantages of being noninvasive and easy to obtain, is under development. The detection period and correlation with impairment are still being established for oral secretion testing (Lee et al. 2011).

Studied Medical Indications for Marijuana Use

Appetite Enhancement in HIV/AIDS

One of the better studied indications for the medical use of marijuana is cachexia, also known as wasting, associated with HIV/AIDS. Indeed, one of the pharmaceutical preparations of THC, dronabinol, has an FDA indication for this purpose. In addition, in an anonymous, cross-sectional, questionnaire-based study of 523 HIV-positive patients, respondents reported that smoking marijuana improved their appetite (Woolridge et al. 2005).

Five small randomized controlled trials (RCTs) have been published specifically examining cannabinoid use for appetite stimulation in HIV/AIDS (see Lutge et al. 2013). Although all of these studies have shown increased caloric intake in individuals using dronabinol or smoking marijuana, only two small studies have demonstrated a statistically significant increase in body weight among individuals randomly assigned to cannabinoid use (Ben Amar 2006; Hazekamp and Grotenhermen 2010).

A Cochrane review of the medical use of marijuana in patients with HIV/ AIDS included seven RCTs of marijuana use of any type (e.g., smoked, oral, dronabinol). The studies were short in duration (21–84 days) and had small sample sizes. The authors also commented on challenges with blinding and on heterogeneity in outcome measures across the studies. They concluded that there was limited evidence for beneficial effects of marijuana in this population. Although the aim of the review was to evaluate whether marijuana reduced morbidity and mortality in HIV patients, the authors noted that the available studies focused on short-term outcome measures only and that there were no studies that examined long-term safety of marijuana or its sustained effects on morbidity or mortality in HIV/AIDS (Lutge et al. 2013).

Pain

Pain is the condition for which medical marijuana is most often recommended and the condition that is the best studied. There are 31 controlled trials of various cannabinoids for neuropathic or chronic pain, including 5 trials involving smoked marijuana (e.g., Ben Amar 2006; Hazekamp and Grotenhermen 2010). These studies showed mixed results, with the majority of studies demonstrating modest reductions in pain, several failing to find a significant difference between cannabinoids and placebo, and 2 showing increases in pain scores with marijuana. One study of neuropathic pain (Wilsey et al. 2008) and 2 studies of HIV-associated sensory neuropathy (Abrams et al. 2007; Ellis et al. 2009) found that marijuana use led to significant decreases in pain (greater than 30% reduction). However, another study of neuropathic pain (Ware et al. 2010) showed a mean reduction of only 0.7 points on a 10-point pain scale in patients with refractory pain. Additionally, a study of experimentally induced neuropathic pain (Wallace et al. 2007) showed significant improvement in analgesia among individuals who smoked marijuana cigarettes containing 4% THC. Interestingly, there was no pain reduction when the marijuana in the cigarette contained only 2% THC, and there was an increase in pain when it contained 8% THC, suggesting that there may be an optimal dosing window. Findings are difficult to generalize to patients with chronic pain because of the short duration of these studies, the small numbers of subjects enrolled (between 15 and 50), the varying THC content of the plant material smoked, and the difficulty of blinding participants to the treatment to which they were randomly assigned. A 2011 systematic review concluded that cannabinoids are modestly effective for the treatment of neuropathic pain (Lynch and Campbell 2011); several authors have likened its effectiveness to that of codeine, a weak opioid analgesic.

A recent systematic review and meta-analysis of cannabinoids for chronic pain analyzed 28 studies and found them to be of low to moderate quality (Whiting et al. 2015). Although these findings suggested improvement in pain with cannabinoids, statistical significance was not achieved in most studies. The researchers' meta-analysis of 8 studies similarly favored cannabinoids over placebo for pain reduction, but the odds of a 30% or greater reduction in pain with cannabinoids did not meet statistical significance. Smaller meta-analyses presented in the same paper found a statistically significant reduction in pain on the Numerical Rating Scale assessment of pain in an analysis of 6 studies of nabiximols, a significant improvement in patients' global impression of change in 6 studies of nabiximols, and a significant reduction in neuropathic pain in an analysis of 5 studies of nabiximols (Whiting et al. 2015).

Spasticity and Multiple Sclerosis

At the time of this writing, more than 20 controlled trials of cannabinoids for muscle spasms and multiple sclerosis (MS)—primarily involving nabiximols, dronabinol, and nabilone—have been conducted. Initial small trials showed mixed efficacy at reducing spasticity. The largest trial on this topic is the Cannabinoids in Multiple Sclerosis (CAMS) study, published in 2003. In this study of 630 patients randomly assigned to taking dronabinol, Cannador (a marijuana extract with THC and CBD similar to nabiximols), or placebo, patients reported subjective decreases in pain, but the investigators were unable to identify an objective improvement in spasticity (Zajicek et al. 2003).

A 2015 systematic review and meta-analysis (Whiting et al. 2015) reviewed 11 studies of cannabinoid use in patients with MS. These studies, which were determined to be of low to moderate quality, generally were associated with improvements in spasticity, but these improvements often failed to reach statistical significance. This meta-analysis was able to pool 5 studies using Cochrane methodology and found that cannabinoids were associated with a greater average improvement on the Ashworth scale for spasticity compared with placebo, but this difference did not reach statistical significance. There were small, statistically significant improvements in spasticity among individuals using cannabinoids in the meta-analysis of 3 studies that used the Numerical Rating Scale and also in the meta-analysis of 3 studies that looked at patients' global impression of change (Whiting et al. 2015).

Nausea

There is evidence that oral formulations of THC are more effective than placebo and are equivalent to traditional antiemetic medications such as prochlorperazine. There have been 32 controlled trials of cannabinoids for nausea, most of which examined chemotherapy-induced nausea and vomiting (Ben Amar 2006; Hazekamp and Grotenhermen 2010). The majority of these studies involved dronabinol or nabilone, but 3 studied smoked marijuana. These small trials had between 8 and 20 subjects and had variable results, with 1 showing no antiemetic effect with a low-dose THC cigarette (Chang et al. 1981), 1 showing improvement in only 25% of subjects (Levitt et al. 1984), and another showing a significant effect over placebo (Chang et al. 1979).

A 2001 systematic review considered studies of dronabinol and nabilone for chemotherapy-associated nausea and vomiting, concluding that cannabinoids were more effective antiemetics than several phenothiazines (e.g., prochlorperazine, metoclopramide, chlorpromazine) but that cannabinoids were more likely to cause adverse effects, including dizziness, dysphoria, and hallucinations (Tramèr et al. 2001). Most of the studies of cannabinoids for nausea and vomiting were done before the availability of serotonin 5-HT$_3$ receptor antagonists such as ondansetron (Zofran), which are generally considered to be more effective than the phenothiazine antiemetics to which cannabinoids had been compared. Although medical marijuana may be effective as an antiemetic, there is no evidence to support its recommendation over modern antiemetic medications, and it is probably most useful in cases of refractory nausea or as an adjuvant therapy.

Seizures

There has been growing interest in the use of marijuana as an antiepileptic, which crescendoed after extensive media reporting surrounding Charlotte Figi, a young girl with a severe form of epilepsy called Dravet syndrome, whose parents noted significant improvement in her symptoms after administering a CBD-predominant extract. At present, 14 American states permit the specific use of CBD extracts for refractory seizures (National Conference of State Legislatures 2015). Outside of these compelling, but anecdotal, reports of efficacy, only small studies are available in the literature. These studies generally indicate that CBD may have promise as a treatment for epilepsy. In a 2013 survey of 19 families using high-CBD strains of marijuana to treat

epileptic seizures in their children, 11% of parents reported complete resolution of seizures, 42% reported a reduction greater than 80% in seizure frequency, and 32% reported a reduction of 25%–60% in seizure frequency
(Porter and Jacobson 2013).

However, there are still scant high-quality data to support the use of cannabinoids in the treatment of epilepsy. A Cochrane review on the subject
found four RCTs with a total of 48 patients, all using CBD. Patients were
continued on their antiepileptic pharmaceuticals. Authors noted that all
studies were of low quality, with small sizes and without descriptions of
blinding. They were not able to draw conclusions about efficacy on the basis
of these studies and were able to conclude only that 200–300 mg/day of CBD
was not found to have adverse effects in the small numbers of patients enrolled for the short duration of the studies (Gloss and Vickrey 2014).

Glaucoma

A handful of small studies have assessed the therapeutic potential of marijuana
as a treatment for glaucoma. In three controlled trials, one using different concentrations of THC-infused eye drops, one with smoked marijuana, and one
with oral marijuana extract, all found that marijuana lowered intraocular pressure (IOP). However, the decrease in IOP with cannabinoids is transient, lasting
several hours only, which would necessitate very frequent marijuana use to con-
tinuously lower IOP (Jampel 2010). In the trial involving smoked marijuana,
almost 44% of patients had tachycardia or palpitations, and another 23% experienced postural hypotension (Merritt et al. 1980). No studies comparing
cannabinoids to current FDA-approved treatments for glaucoma are available. In 2010, the American Glaucoma Society issued a position statement
that concluded, "Although marijuana can lower the IOP, its side effects and
short duration of action, coupled with a lack of evidence that it shortens the
course of glaucoma, preclude recommending this drug in any form for the
treatment of glaucoma at the present time" (Jampel 2010, p. 76).

Hepatitis C

Hepatitis C virus (HCV) infection is an approved indication for medical
marijuana use in some states, largely because of a small 2006 RCT that investigated the effects of marijuana use in patients undergoing treatment for
HCV. In the study, marijuana users were found to have better adherence to
their HCV treatment and resultant higher rates of sustained virologic response to treatment than nonusers (Sylvestre et al. 2006). In addition, multiple studies have investigated the role of the endocannabinoid system in
hepatic fibrogenesis in patients with chronic hepatitis C. In a prospective co-

hort study of 204 people with HCV, daily marijuana use was identified as an independent risk factor for moderate to severe fibrosis, with marijuana users having a nearly sevenfold higher odds of moderate to severe fibrosis compared with nondaily users (Ishida et al. 2008). Another study found that daily marijuana smoking is an independent predictor of steatosis severity, which is itself an independent predictor of liver fibrosis in chronic hepatitis C patients (Hézode et al. 2008). Although marijuana use may help patients manage the adverse effects of HCV treatment, and therefore increase treatment adherence, the associations between marijuana use and higher rates of hepatic fibrosis suggest that we should discourage HCV-infected patients from marijuana use. Curative treatments for HCV will likely obviate the need for considering medical marijuana for this condition.

Crohn's Disease

Marijuana has been used to treat multiple gastrointestinal disorders, including pain, nausea, anorexia, diarrhea, gastroenteritis, diabetic gastroparesis, and inflammation (Naftali et al. 2013). There has also been anecdotal evidence suggesting possible benefit of inhaled marijuana in Crohn's disease, as well as research supporting a mediating role of the endocannabinoid system in colonic inflammation (Wright et al. 2008). Small observational studies have shown reductions in disease activity when marijuana is used with other medications, but studies have been limited by small samples, short durations, and subjective outcomes. In the only controlled trial of marijuana in Crohn's disease, 21 patients were randomly assigned to treatment with smoked marijuana or placebo. Those in the intervention group had significant increases in quality of life, improved appetite, less pain, and higher treatment satisfaction compared with the placebo group. There were no notable differences in side effects between the two groups. Although the trial found that 50% of patients in the study achieved induction of remission on subjective symptomatic scales as defined by the Crohn's Disease Activity Index, there was no objective evidence of reduction in inflammation. Patients in the study also relapsed within 2 weeks of stopping marijuana treatment. On the basis of these findings, the authors of the study recommended marijuana for compassionate use in patients with Crohn's disease who had exhausted medical and surgical options but discouraged its use as a primary treatment (Naftali et al. 2013).

Amyotrophic Lateral Sclerosis

Amyotrophic lateral sclerosis (ALS) is an approved indication for medical marijuana use in several states. ALS is a devastating disease for which no disease-altering treatments exist, but there is interest in cannabinoids as treatment agents because cannabinoid receptors are expressed on immune cells and likely help regulate the immune system. In addition, endogenous cannabinoids seem to down-regulate cytokine and chemokine production, thus suppressing inflammatory responses. Since neuroinflammation and immune dysregulation appear to have a role in ALS, cannabinoids are intriguing potential treatment agents. Further, mouse models have suggested involvement of the endocannabinoid system in the pathophysiology of the disease and have also shown slower progression of disease with synthetic cannabinoids. To date, these animal model findings have not been translated into a disease-altering treatment for ALS in humans (Carter et al. 2010). In a 2004 survey of 13 ALS patients who used marijuana, respondents reported modest reductions in depression, drooling, pain, spasticity, and appetite loss (Amtmann et al. 2004). There are no published controlled trials of marijuana in this patient population.

Dementia

As discussed in the previous subsection with regard to ALS, cannabinoids seem to have immunomodulatory and anti-inflammatory properties, so there is interest in cannabinoid treatment as a means of decreasing symptoms and potentially altering the course of neurodegenerative conditions, including dementia. Altered components of the endocannabinoid system have been found in the brains of deceased Alzheimer's patients, including increased expression of cannabinoid receptors on microglia in senile plaques and up-regulation of endocannabinoid metabolizing enzymes, which may contribute to neuroinflammation. These changes suggest that the endocannabinoid system may be involved in the pathophysiology of Alzheimer's dementia (Campbell and Gowran 2007). A retrospective study of 40 patients found that total agitation scores on the Pittsburgh Agitation Scale decreased significantly during dronabinol treatment at a mean dose of 7.0 mg/day for an average of 16.9 days and that individual Pittsburgh Agitation Scale domain scores also showed improvements (Woodward et al. 2014). This study noted a significant decrease in resisting care, a significant increase in percentage of food consumed at each meal, and significant improvements in Clinical Global Impression Scale scores.

There has been only one RCT of cannabinoids for symptom management in dementia. This study of dronabinol included 15 patients and found increases in body weight and decreases in disturbed behavior in patients receiving dronabinol (Volicer et al. 1997). Although these initial findings are promising, a Cochrane review of cannabinoids for dementia noted that the RCT by Volicer and colleagues did not provide sufficient data from which to draw useful conclusions and indicated that there was no evidence that cannabinoids are effective in the treatment of behavioral disturbances associated with dementia (Krishnan et al. 2009).

Parkinson's Disease

There is evidence in animal models to suggest that marijuana, particularly CBD, may be helpful in the treatment of Parkinson's disease. A study of CBD in six patients with Parkinson's suggested improvement in overall Parkinson's symptoms and psychosis (Zuardi et al. 2009). One controlled trial of marijuana in Parkinson's disease in humans did not show improvement in motor and symptom scores but did show significant improvements in quality-of-life scores (Chagas et al. 2014).

Psychiatric Conditions and Medical Marijuana

Psychosis

Marijuana can induce psychotic symptoms in otherwise healthy volunteers, persons at risk for psychotic disorders, and patients with schizophrenia. The etiology of this association remains poorly elucidated, but it appears to be related to high-potency THC exposure. In contrast, there is preliminary evidence that CBD has antipsychotic properties (Schubart et al. 2014). In a Phase II 28-day trial of 42 persons with schizophrenia experiencing acute psychosis who were randomly assigned to receive either 800 mg of amisulpride or 800 mg of CBD, subjects given amisulpride and subjects given CBD both experienced significant clinical improvement, but subjects given CBD had a lower incidence of adverse effects (Leweke et al. 2012). However, when the authors of a recent meta-analysis examined these studies using the Cochrane Collaboration's Risk of Bias Tool, a global measure of systematic error, they found these studies to be at high risk of bias (Whiting et al. 2015), so using CBD to treat persons with schizophrenia remains only a potential treatment.

A Cochrane review of marijuana and schizophrenia concluded that current evidence is insufficient to show if the antipsychotic effects of CBD are equivalent to those of conventional treatments in nonrefractory schizophrenia (McLoughlin et al. 2014). Although CBD remains an experimental treatment, the risks of using currently available marijuana, which is often high in THC, for persons with psychotic disorders are well characterized. Heavy marijuana use, high potency of consumed marijuana, and younger age at initiation of use have been tied to worsened disease trajectories and advancing the time of a first psychotic episode in vulnerable people by as much as 2–6 years (Volkow et al. 2014). Although there may be a future role for CBD in treatment-refractory psychosis and in patients who cannot tolerate conventional antipsychotics, the association between marijuana use and psychosis makes marijuana use, especially strains with high THC:CBD ratios, inadvisable among persons with, or at risk for developing, psychotic disorders.

Mania

Patients with mood disorders, such as Jacob in the opening clinical vignette, may dislike conventional medications and their potential adverse effects and instead prefer to use a "natural" or "alternative" treatment. The available evidence, however, does not support using marijuana in the treatment of persons with bipolar disorder. A 2010 trial showed no improvement in symptoms with CBD monotherapy dosed from 600 to 1,200 mg daily (Zuardi et al. 2010). Review of existing literature reveals an association between marijuana use and exacerbations of manic symptoms in patients previously diagnosed with bipolar disorder, including the prevalence, duration, and severity of manic episodes (Gibbs et al. 2015). In a 2-year prospective observational study of 1,922 adults with bipolar disorder, patients who reported marijuana use experienced an earlier age at onset of bipolar disorder along with more manic episodes, hospitalizations, and suicide attempts. These patients also reported poorer functional outcomes. In this study, the striking finding is that 2 years after cessation, patients with bipolar disorder who discontinued marijuana use had similar clinical and functional outcomes to those who had never used marijuana (Zorrilla et al. 2015). Given this evidence, health care providers should discourage marijuana use among patients with bipolar disorder.

Depression

Evidence from longitudinal studies investigating the role that marijuana use plays in depression is mixed, but many investigators have found that regular marijuana use predicts a modestly increased risk of subsequent depressive episodes (van Laar et al. 2007). The risks appear most profound if marijuana use begins in adolescence. For example, in a longitudinal survey that followed 2,033 adolescents in Norway over a 13-year period, using marijuana more than 11 times in the past 12 months was associated with significantly increased risk of suicidal ideation and suicide attempts when subjects were in their 20s (Pedersen 2008). In a recent meta-analysis of the associations between marijuana use and depression, the authors found a dose effect, concluding that heavy, habitual marijuana use is associated with an increased risk of depression (Lev-Ran et al. 2014).

Anxiety

Jacob reported that marijuana use reduced not only his insomnia but his anxiety as well. Subjectively decreasing anxiety is a common reason for using marijuana as a medical treatment, but a recent meta-analysis found that although cannabinoids may be superior to placebo in reducing anxiety symptoms, the available trials are so small and at risk for bias, when evaluated using the Cochrane Risk of Bias Tool, that the authors believed no conclusions could be made (Whiting et al. 2015). Some short-duration trials have found that CBD and nabilone were useful at doses of 300–600 mg and 2–5 mg, respectively, but others have found that marijuana, particularly with THC concentrations greater than 5 mg, could induce intense fear, panic attacks, and short-lived anxiety episodes in nonhabitual users (Crippa et al. 2009).

Formulations with high THC:CBD ratios appear to increase scores on anxiety scales, and those with low THC:CBD ratios often decrease scores on anxiety scales. Indeed, functional magnetic resonance imaging studies show that when subjects view fearful stimuli, CBD modulates brain activity patterns by attenuating responses in the anterior and posterior cingulate cortex and in the amygdala and acts on prefrontal subcortical pathways through the anterior cingulate cortex and amygdala to produce anxiolytic effects (Crippa et al. 2010). These findings are in accord with animal models that suggest that low doses of CBD have anxiolytic properties through interaction with 5-HT_{1A} receptors rather than γ-aminobutyric acid receptors (Crippa et al. 2010). Among human studies, this suggestive finding is supported by a small randomized trial in which 300 mg of CBD in healthy subjects improved the anxiety induced by simulated public speaking in a manner comparable to 5 mg of ipsapirone, a selective 5-HT_{1A} receptor partial agonist (Zuardi et al. 1993). In social anxiety disorder specifically, 600 mg of CBD decreased anxiety scores on the visual analogue scale after public speaking, and 300 mg attenuated anxiety in healthy volunteers (Schier et al. 2012). CBD is noted to have a U-shaped curve of effect with no anxiolytic effects in doses >100 mg/kg but decreased THC-induced conditioned emotional responses at 10 mg/kg. Nabilone at doses of 2–5 mg has been shown to reduce symptoms on the Hamilton Anxiety Scale and, in a study of patients with anxiety disorders, to reduce symptoms after 28 days of treatment (Crippa et al. 2009). However, generalizability is limited because most of these trials had a small number of subjects and a brief duration of treatment and primarily enrolled healthy subjects.

Posttraumatic Stress Disorder

The associations between marijuana use and posttraumatic stress disorder (PTSD) are complex. Groups with high rates of PTSD report high rates of marijuana use (Bonn-Miller et al. 2012), and the National Comorbidity Survey found that adults with PTSD were three times more likely to experience cannabis dependence than adults without PTSD (Cornelius et al. 2010). However, it is not clear whether marijuana causes, exacerbates, or even alleviates some of the many symptoms of PTSD. The core symptom of PTSD, the consolidation of traumatic memories, is facilitated by glucocorticoid hormones that potentiate norepinephrine in the basolateral amygdala. Because cannabinoid receptors mediate the action of glucocorticoid hormones, there are compelling scientific reasons to study the relationships between marijuana use and PTSD. At some point, targeted modulation of the cannabinoid type 1 receptor in the central nervous system may be a treatment strategy for PTSD. At present, most of this work is being conducted through animal models and imaging studies (Neumeister et al. 2013). A recent review of the subject observed that no randomized trials of marijuana for PTSD have been conducted and that sufficient evidence is lacking to recommend the use of marijuana for PTSD at present (Belendiuk et al. 2015). Meanwhile, marijuana use by persons with PTSD is known to exacerbate impairments in memory, attention, concentration, and information processing (Borgelt et al. 2013).

Sleep-Wake Disturbances

Like Jacob, patients often present to a practitioner's office reporting that they use marijuana to help initiate and maintain sleep. CBD has been evaluated and found to have a biphasic effect in which low doses induced wakefulness and high doses led to sedation. In a small study of healthy subjects, 15 mg doses of CBD increased wakefulness, possibly by increasing dopamine levels (Zuardi 2008). In other studies, nabilone has been found to improve sleep in fibromyalgia patients (Crippa et al. 2010). Nabiximols was found to improve subjective sleep parameters when used to treat spasticity and pain, but it probably does not significantly impact sleep architecture (Gates et al. 2014).

A 2014 systematic review of the effects of cannabinoids on sleep concluded that recreational marijuana use could lead to interrupted sleep cycles and leave the user with the impression of ineffective sleep even though the number of nighttime awakenings and amount of time spent asleep are not affected. Medical marijuana use, on the other hand, seems to show reduced sleep disturbances with subjective improvements in sleep. The authors noted that in patients using marijuana for chronic medical conditions (e.g., pain), cannabinoids may alleviate the symptoms of those medical conditions and thus decrease sleep disruption. The authors noted that most studies in the systematic review were of low quality and short duration and resulted in mixed findings. They were often limited by methodological issues, including lack of validated sleep measures or objective observation (Gates et al. 2014).

Adverse Effects

Although marijuana is sometimes thought of as having few or no adverse effects, there are well documented adverse effects of marijuana use, as outlined in Table 4–4.

TABLE 4–4.   Adverse effects of marijuana use

Adverse effects associated with short-term marijuana use

1. Impaired short-term memory and impaired ability to learn and retain information

2. Impaired motor coordination leading to increased risk of injuries

3. Altered judgment with possible increase in high-risk sexual behavior and increased risk of sexually transmitted infections

4. Paranoia

5. Psychosis

6. Immunosuppression

Adverse effects associated with long-term or heavy marijuana use

1. Addiction: 9.1% of overall users, 17% of those who begin use in adolescence, and 25%–50% of daily users

2. Chronic bronchitis symptoms

3. Increased risk of psychotic disorders, including schizophrenia, in persons with predisposition to such disorders

Adverse effects associated with long-term or heavy marijuana use with initial use in early adolescence

1. Altered brain development (changes in size, shape, and density of parts of the brain, especially the amygdala and nucleus accumbens)

2. Poor educational attainment with increased likelihood of school dropout

3. Cognitive impairment/lower IQ

4. Diminished life satisfaction and achievement

5. Cardiovascular effects, including tachycardia and postural hypotension

6. Decreased sperm counts

Source.   Croxford 2003; Volkow et al. 2014.

Effects in Pregnancy and Lactation

Because the key cannabinoids are highly lipophilic, they are able to cross the placenta to the fetus and can be detected in the umbilical cord blood and urine of neonates born to marijuana users (Hill and Reed 2013). Studying the impact of this marijuana exposure in neonates and children who were exposed in utero is challenging because women who use marijuana are more likely to smoke tobacco and use other drugs, have a mental illness, live in poverty, and have poor nutrition compared with their counterparts who do not use marijuana (Jaques et al. 2014). Separating the effects of marijuana on an infant or child from the effects of the other factors is difficult, particularly because most cohort studies rely on self-reporting of marijuana use, which has potential reporting and recall bias.

Studies of the effects of marijuana use in pregnancy have yielded conflicting results, with some finding an association between marijuana use and preterm birth, stillbirth, low birth weight, and neonatal intensive care admission and others finding no differences between infants born to mothers who used marijuana and those who did not (Mark et al. 2015). When cohorts of children are followed through an older age, there are again conflicting results, with some studies suggesting increased impulsivity and decreased attention in early childhood and cognitive changes, particularly in executive function, in adolescence. Other cohort studies did not find significant differences between the groups. No studies found significant differences in IQ (Hill and Reed 2013).

There are no high-quality studies of the effects on an infant breastfeeding from a mother who uses marijuana. Marijuana is also transferred into breast milk, but sources disagree on the concentration of THC in breast milk, with some studies reporting lower concentrations in milk compared with the mother's blood and others reporting up to an eightfold increase in THC concentration in breast milk compared with maternal blood samples (Djulus et al. 2005). One small cohort study reported decreased motor development at age 1 year in children of mothers who had used marijuana while breastfeeding (Astley and Little 1990), but this finding has not been corroborated. The American Academy of Pediatrics (Section on Breastfeeding 2012) considers maternal marijuana use to be a contraindication to breastfeeding. A position statement by the American College of Obstetricians and Gynecologists' Committee on Obstetric Practice (2015) similarly recommended that women who are pregnant or contemplating pregnancy should be encouraged to discontinue marijuana use and that in the absence of data on marijuana use in lactation, marijuana use is discouraged during breastfeeding.

Marijuana-Medication Interactions

Interactions between marijuana and pharmaceuticals generally consist of elevated levels of the other drugs. This includes anticoagulant and antiplatelet medications, anesthetic agents, chemotherapy agents, barbiturates, antiviral medications, and some antibiotics. Marijuana can also induce hypomania when used together with some antidepressant medications and is synergistic when mixed with alcohol and other central nervous system depressants. Specific mechanisms and medications are listed in Table 4–5.

TABLE 4–5.   Marijuana-medication interactions

Mechanism	Drugs
1. Inhibition of platelet aggregation: THC/CBD may increase risk of bleeding when used with anticoagulant and antiplatelet drugs	Nonsteroidal anti-inflammatory drugs: diclofenac, ibuprofen, naproxen Anticoagulants: clopidogrel, dalteparin, enoxaparin, heparin, warfarin[a]
2. Competition with barbiturate metabolism → increased drug levels	Pentobarbital, phenobarbital, secobarbital
3. Antiestrogenic effects	Contraceptive drugs Estrogens/hormone therapy
4. Cytochrome P450 2E1 (CYP2E1) induction → decreased levels of drugs metabolized by CYP2E1	Acetaminophen, chlorzoxazone, ethanol, theophylline, anesthetics (enflurane, halothane, isoflurane, methoxyflurane)
5. Cytochrome P450 3A4 (CYP3A4) inhibition → increased levels of drugs metabolized by CYP3A4	Lovastatin, clarithromycin, cyclosporine, diltiazem, estrogens, indinavir, triazolam
6. Inhibition of P-glycoproteins (CBD/THC) → increased levels of substrates	Chemotherapy agents: etoposide, paclitaxel, vinblastine, vincristine, vindesine Antifungals: ketoconazole, itraconazole Protease inhibitors: amprenavir, indinavir, nelfinavir, saquinavir Histamine H_2 antagonists: cimetidine, ranitidine Calcium channel blockers: diltiazem, verapamil Others: corticosteroids, erythromycin, cisapride, fexofenadine, cyclosporine, quinidine, loperamide
7. Increased metabolism of theophylline	Theophylline
8. Additive/synergistic effects	Alcohol Central nervous system depressants
9. Induction of hypomania	Fluoxetine Disulfiram

Note.   CBD=cannabidiol; THC=Δ^9-tetrahydrocannabinol.
[a]Decreased warfarin metabolism or decreased amount bound to plasma proteins results in increased warfarin effects and elevated international normalized ratio.
Source.   Natural Medicines Comprehensive Database 2015.

Key Points

- As more states adopt legislation permitting medical and recreational use of marijuana, it is important for mental health professionals to understand the formulations and routes of administration of marijuana.

- Several pharmaceutical formulations of marijuana are available or under development in the United States and abroad. Dronabinol (marketed as Marinol) and nabilone (marketed as Cesamet) are FDA approved in the United States for the treatment of chemotherapy-induced nausea and vomiting; dronabinol is, additionally, approved for AIDS-associated anorexia.

- The marijuana plant contains at least 70 known cannabinoids, the best known and understood of which is THC. Others, particularly CBD, are being investigated for medicinal properties.

- An extensive list of medical indications for marijuana use has been studied, with HIV/AIDS-induced anorexia and weight loss, pain, chemotherapy-induced nausea and vomiting, and spasticity being the most frequently studied conditions. The most promising evidence pertains to pain, nausea, and spasticity. Qualifying indications for medical marijuana use vary across states. At present, the evidence for the medical use of marijuana remains preliminary. In addition, most research has been conducted on formulations that are of lower potency than the formulations available in dispensaries, so it is difficult to extrapolate from the limited scientific literature to contemporary formulations.

- Increasing research is being conducted on possible psychiatric indications for marijuana use. Evidence has been conflicting for benefit in disorders such as anxiety disorders and PTSD. There is strong evidence that marijuana use exacerbates many other disorders, including depression, bipolar disorder, and psychotic disorders. The use of CBD for the treatment of psychosis warrants further investigation.

- A variety of both short- and long-term adverse effects from marijuana use have been elucidated, and there is particular concern about adverse effects when use begins in adolescence. Common short-term effects are paranoia; psychosis; and impaired motor functioning, judgment, and memory. Long-term effects include addiction, respiratory disorders, and increased risk of a psychotic disorder in susceptible individuals. Long-term effects related to adolescent use include impaired cognition and decreased IQ, as well as poor educational outcomes.

References

Abrams DI, Jay CA, Shade SB, et al: Cannabis in painful HIV-associated sensory neuropathy: a randomized placebo-controlled trial. Neurology 68(7):515–521, 2007 17296917

American College of Obstetricians and Gynecologists Committee on Obstetric Practice: Committee opinion no. 637: marijuana use during pregnancy and lactation. Obstet Gynecol 126(1):234–238, 2015 26241291

Americans for Safe Access: Guide to Using Medical Cannabis. Oakland, CA, Americans for Safe Access, 2015. Available at: http://www.safeaccessnow.org/using_medical_cannabis. Accessed May 30, 2015.

Amtmann D, Weydt P, Johnson KL, et al: Survey of cannabis use in patients with amyotrophic lateral sclerosis. Am J Hosp Palliat Care 21(2):95–104, 2004 15055508

Astley SJ, Little RE: Maternal marijuana use during lactation and infant development at one year. Neurotoxicol Teratol 12(2):161–168, 1990 2333069

Baca R: More than 15 months in, pot-infused edibles still confound. The Denver Post, April 12, 2015. Available at: http://www.denverpost.com/news/ci_27896734/report-more-than-15-months-pot-infused-edibles. Accessed April 15, 2015.

Belendiuk KA, Baldini LL, Bonn-Miller MO: Narrative review of the safety and efficacy of marijuana for the treatment of commonly state-approved medical and psychiatric disorders. Addict Sci Clin Pract 10(1):10, 2015 25896576

Ben Amar M: Cannabinoids in medicine: a review of their therapeutic potential. J Ethnopharmacol 105(1–2):1–25, 2006 16540272

Bonn-Miller MO, Harris AH, Trafton JA: Prevalence of cannabis use disorder diagnoses among veterans in 2002, 2008, and 2009. Psychol Serv 9(4):404–416, 2012 22564034

Borgelt LM, Franson KL, Nussbaum AM, et al: The pharmacologic and clinical effects of medical cannabis. Pharmacotherapy 33(2):195–209, 2013 23386598

Brohl B, Kammerzell R, Koski WL: Colorado Marijuana Enforcement Division Annual Update. Denver, Colorado Department of Revenue, February 27, 2015

Burns TL, Ineck JR: Cannabinoid analgesia as a potential new therapeutic option in the treatment of chronic pain. Ann Pharmacother 40(2):251–260, 2006 16449552

Campbell VA, Gowran A: Alzheimer's disease; taking the edge off with cannabinoids? Br J Pharmacol 152(5):655–662, 2007 17828287

Carter GT, Abood ME, Aggarwal SK, et al: Cannabis and amyotrophic lateral sclerosis: hypothetical and practical applications, and a call for clinical trials. Am J Hosp Palliat Care 27(5):347–356, 2010 20439484

Chagas MH, Zuardi AW, Tumas V, et al: Effects of cannabidiol in the treatment of patients with Parkinson's disease: an exploratory double-blind trial. J Psychopharmacol 28(11):1088–1098, 2014 25237116

Chang AE, Shiling DJ, Stillman RC, et al: Delta-9-tetrahydrocannabinol as an antiemetic in cancer patients receiving high-dose methotrexate: a prospective, randomized evaluation. Ann Intern Med 91(6):819–824, 1979 293141

Chang AE, Shiling DJ, Stillman RC, et al: A prospective evaluation of delta-9-tetra-hydrocannabinol as an antiemetic in patients receiving Adriamycin and Cy-toxan chemotherapy. Cancer 47(7):1746–1751, 1981

Cornelius JR, Kirisci L, Reynolds M, et al: PTSD contributes to teen and young adult cannabis use disorders. Addict Behav 35(2):91–94, 2010 19773127

Crippa JA, Zuardi AW, Martín-Santos R, et al: Cannabis and anxiety: a critical review of the evidence. Hum Psychopharmacol 24(7):515–523, 2009 19693792

Crippa JA, Zuardi AW, Hallak JE: Therapeutical use of the cannabinoids in psychia-try [in Portuguese]. J Rev Bras Psiquiatr 32 (suppl 1):S56–S66, 2010 20512271

Croxford JL: Therapeutic potential of cannabinoids in CNS disease. CNS Drugs 17(3):179–202, 2003 12617697

Djulus J, Moretti M, Koren G: Marijuana use and breastfeeding. Can Fam Physician 51:349–350, 2005 15794018

Ellis RJ, Toperoff W, Vaida F, et al: Smoked medicinal cannabis for neuropathic pain in HIV: a randomized, crossover clinical trial. Neuropsychopharmacology 34(3):672–680, 2009 18688212

Gates PJ, Albertella L, Copeland J: The effects of cannabinoid administration on sleep: a systematic review of human studies. Sleep Med Rev 18(6):477–487, 2014 24726015

Gibbs M, Winsper C, Marwaha S, et al: Cannabis use and mania symptoms: a system-atic review and meta-analysis. J Affect Disord 171:39–47, 2015 25285897

Gloss D, Vickrey B: Cannabinoids for epilepsy. Cochrane Database Syst Rev (3):CD009270, 2014

Grotenhermen F: Pharmacokinetics and pharmacodynamics of cannabinoids. Clin Pharmacokinet 42(4):327–360, 2003 12648025

Hartman RL, Huestis MA: Cannabis effects on driving skills. Clin Chem 59(3):478–492, 2013 23220273

Hazekamp A, Grotenhermen F: Review on clinical studies with cannabis and canna-binoids 2005–2009. Cannabinoids 5(special issue):1–21, 2010

Hézode C, Zafrani ES, Roudot-Thoraval F, et al: Daily cannabis use: a novel risk fac-tor of steatosis severity in patients with chronic hepatitis C. Gastroenterology 134(2):432–439, 2008 18242211

Hill M, Reed K: Pregnancy, breast-feeding, and marijuana: a review article. Obstet Gy-necol Surv 68(10):710–718, 2013 25101905

Huestis MA: Human cannabinoid pharmacokinetics. Chem Biodivers 4(8):1770–1804, 2007 17712819

Ishida JH, Peters MG, Jin C, et al: Influence of cannabis use on severity of hepatitis C disease. Clin Gastroenterol Hepatol 6(1):69–75, 2008 18166478

Jampel H: American Glaucoma Society position statement: marijuana and the treat-ment of glaucoma. J Glaucoma 19(2):75–76, 2010 20160576

Jaques SC, Kingsbury A, Henshcke P, et al: Cannabis, the pregnant woman and her child: weeding out the myths. J Perinatol 34(6):417–424, 2014 24457255

Krishnan S, Cairns R, Howard R: Cannabinoids for the treatment of dementia. Cochrane Database Syst Rev (2):CD007204, 2009 19370677

Lee D, Milman G, Barnes AJ, et al: Oral fluid cannabinoids in chronic, daily cannabis smokers during sustained, monitored abstinence. Clin Chem 57(8):1127–1136, 2011 21677094

Levitt M, Faiman C, Hawks R, et al: Randomized double-blind comparison of delta-9-tetrahydrocannabinol (THC) and marijuana as chemotherapy antiemetics. Proc Am Soc Clin Oncol 3:91, 1984

Lev-Ran S, Roerecke M, Le Foll B, et al: The association between cannabis use and depression: a systematic review and meta-analysis of longitudinal studies. Psychol Med 44(4):797–810, 2014 23795762

Leweke FM, Piomelli D, Pahlisch F, et al: Cannabidiol enhances anandamide signaling and alleviates psychotic symptoms of schizophrenia. Transl Psychiatry 2(3):e94, 2012 22832859

Lutge EE, Gray A, Siegfried N: The medical use of cannabis for reducing morbidity and mortality in patients with HIV/AIDS. Cochrane Database Syst Rev 4(4):CD005175, 2013 23633327

Lynch ME, Campbell F: Cannabinoids for treatment of chronic non-cancer pain; a systematic review of randomized trials. Br J Clin Pharmacol 72(5):735–744, 2011 21426373

Mark K, Desai A, Terplan M: Marijuana use and pregnancy: prevalence, associated characteristics, and birth outcomes. Arch Womens Ment Health, April 29, 2005 25895138 [Epub ahead of print]

McLaren J, Swift W, Dillon P, et al: Cannabis potency and contamination: a review of the literature. Addiction 103(7):1100–1109, 2008 18494838

McLoughlin BC, Pushpa-Rajah JA, Gillies D, et al: Cannabis and schizophrenia. Cochrane Database Syst Rev 10(10):CD004837, 2014 25314586

Merritt JC, Crawford WJ, Alexander PC, et al: Effect of marihuana on intraocular and blood pressure in glaucoma. Ophthalmology 87(3):222–228, 1980 7053160

Naftali T, Bar-Lev Schleider L, Dotan I, et al: Cannabis induces a clinical response in patients with Crohn's disease: a prospective placebo-controlled study. Clin Gastroenterol Hepatol 11(10):1276–1280.e1, 2013 23648372

National Conference of State Legislatures: State Medical Marijuana Laws. Washington, DC, National Conference of State Legislatures, May 12, 2015. Available at: http://www.ncsl.org/research/health/state-medical-marijuana-laws.aspx#3. Accessed August 15, 2015.

Natural Medicines Comprehensive Database: Marijuana. Stockton, CA, Therapeutic Research Faculty. Available at: http://naturaldatabase.therapeuticresearch.com/nd/Search.aspx?pt=100&id=947. Accessed November 16, 2015.

Neumeister A, Normandin MD, Pietrzak RH, et al: Elevated brain cannabinoid CB1 receptor availability in post-traumatic stress disorder: a positron emission tomography study. Mol Psychiatry 18(9):1034–1040, 2013 23670490

Ohlsson A, Lindgren JE, Wahlen A, et al: Plasma delta-9 tetrahydrocannabinol concentrations and clinical effects after oral and intravenous administration and smoking. Clin Pharmacol Ther 28(3):409–416, 1980 6250760

Pearce DD, Mitsouras K, Irizarry KJ: Discriminating the effects of Cannabis sativa and Cannabis indica: a web survey of medical cannabis users. J Altern Complement Med 20(10):787–791, 2014 25191852

Pedersen W: Does cannabis use lead to depression and suicidal behaviours? A population-based longitudinal study. Acta Psychiatr Scand 118(5):395–403, 2008 18798834

Phan HM, Yoshizuka K, Murry DJ, et al: Drug testing in the workplace. Pharmacotherapy 32(7):649–656, 2012 22605533

Porter BE, Jacobson C: Report of a parent survey of cannabidiol-enriched cannabis use in pediatric treatment-resistant epilepsy. Epilepsy Behav 29(3):574–577, 2013 24237632

Schier AR, Ribeiro NP, Silva AC, et al: Cannabidiol, a Cannabis sativa constituent, as an anxiolytic drug. Rev Bras Psiquiatr 34 (suppl 1):S104–S110, 2012 22729452

Schubart CD, Sommer IE, Fusar-Poli P, et al: Cannabidiol as a potential treatment for psychosis. Eur Neuropsychopharmacol 24(1):51–64, 2014 24309088

Section on Breastfeeding: Breastfeeding and the use of human milk. Pediatrics 129(3):e827–e841, 2012 22371471

Sylvestre DL, Clements BJ, Malibu Y: Cannabis use improves retention and virological outcomes in patients treated for hepatitis C. Eur J Gastroenterol Hepatol 18(10):1057–1063, 2006 16957511

Tramèr MR, Carroll D, Campbell FA, et al: Cannabinoids for control of chemotherapy induced nausea and vomiting: quantitative systematic review. BMJ 323(7303):16–21, 2001 11440936

van Laar M, van Dorsselaer S, Monshouwer K, de Graaf R: Does cannabis use predict the first incidence of mood and anxiety disorders in the adult population? Addiction 102(8):1251–1260, 2007 17624975

Volicer L, Stelly M, Morris J, et al: Effects of dronabinol on anorexia and disturbed behavior in patients with Alzheimer's disease. Int J Geriatr Psychiatry 12(9):913–919, 1997 9309469

Volkow ND, Baler RD, Compton WM, et al: Adverse health effects of marijuana use. N Engl J Med 370(23):2219–2227, 2014 24897085

Wallace M, Schulteis G, Atkinson JH, et al: Dose-dependent effects of smoked cannabis on capsaicin-induced pain and hyperalgesia in healthy volunteers. Anesthesiology 107(5):785–796, 2007 18073554

Ware MA, Wang T, Shapiro S, et al: Smoked cannabis for chronic neuropathic pain: a randomized controlled trial. CMAJ 182(14):E694–E701, 2010 20805210

Whiting PF, Wolff RF, Deshpande S, et al: Cannabinoids for medical use: a systematic review and meta-analysis. JAMA 313(24):2456–2473, 2015 26103030

Wilsey B, Marcotte T, Tsodikov A, et al: A randomized, placebo-controlled, crossover trial of cannabis cigarettes in neuropathic pain. J Pain 9(6):506–521, 2008 18403272

Woodward MR, Harper DG, Stolyar A, et al: Dronabinol for the treatment of agitation and aggressive behavior in acutely hospitalized severely demented patients with noncognitive behavioral symptoms. Am J Geriatr Psychiatry 22(4):415–419, 2014 23597932

Woolridge E, Barton S, Samuel J, et al: Cannabis use in HIV for pain and other medical symptoms. J Pain Symptom Manage 29(4):358–367, 2005 15857739

Wright KL, Duncan M, Sharkey KA: Cannabinoid CB2 receptors in the gastrointestinal tract: a regulatory system in states of inflammation. Br J Pharmacol 153(2):263–270, 2008 17906675

Zajicek J, Fox P, Sanders H, et al: Cannabinoids for treatment of spasticity and other symptoms related to multiple sclerosis (CAMS study): multicentre randomised placebo-controlled trial. Lancet 362(9395):1517–1526, 2003 14615106

Zorrilla I, Aguado J, Haro JM, et al: Cannabis and bipolar disorder: does quitting cannabis use during manic/mixed episode improve clinical/functional outcomes? Acta Psychiatr Scand 131(2):100–110, 2015 25430820

Zuardi AW: Cannabidiol: from an inactive cannabinoid to a drug with wide spectrum of action. Rev Bras Psiquiatr 30(3):271–280, 2008 18833429

Zuardi AW, Cosme RA, Graeff FG, et al: Effects of ipsapirone and cannabidiol on human experimental anxiety. J Psychopharmacol 7(1 suppl):82–88, 1993 22290374

Zuardi AW, Crippa JA, Hallak JE, et al: Cannabidiol for the treatment of psychosis in Parkinson's disease. J Psychopharmacol 23(8):979–983, 2009 18801821

Zuardi A, Crippa J, Dursun S, et al: Cannabidiol was ineffective for manic episode of bipolar affective disorder. J Psychopharmacol 24(1):135–137, 2010 18801823

Marijuana Use and Comorbidity

Risk for Substance Use Disorders and Associations With Mood, Anxiety, and Other Behavioral Health Disorders

Charles Luther, M.D.

Matthew Lorber, M.D., M.P.A.

Ruth S. Shim, M.D., M.P.H.

Clinical Vignette: Bryan and His Parents

Bryan Camellia is a 14-year-old high school freshman who has been previously treated for attention-deficit/hyperactivity disorder (ADHD). His teachers have recently noticed worsening problems with attention and classroom participation. Furthermore, Bryan's English teacher, Mr. Donald Lively, has noticed that he is increasingly melancholic and has made nihilistic statements. Mr. Lively is concerned for Bryan's safety and refers him to the school nurse, who calls 911 after Bryan states, "I'd be better off dead." He is taken to the local emergency department, where his evaluation reveals minimal suicide risk but symptoms of depressed mood, excessive worry, and insomnia. A drug screen is obtained and is found to be positive for marijuana. The emergency department physician refers Bryan for immediate follow-up at the local adolescent mental health clinic.

Jon and Amanda, Bryan's parents, accompany Bryan to the clinic the next day for an initial appointment with Dr. Hope Saunders, a child and adolescent psychiatrist. On examination, she notes that Bryan appears anxious, dysphoric, and reluctant to engage in a discussion of his problems and goals. With time and an empathic approach, Dr. Saunders encourages Bryan to share that his father forbids his marijuana use because of "fears that I'll be-

come a drug addict," although his mother espouses a more permissive attitude. Bryan feels his marijuana use helps him sleep and alleviates anxiety; it
helps "loosen me up" when hanging out with friends. However, he is worried
that it may lead to "long-term problems." He acknowledges that he feels depressed for days at a time and that marijuana helps to elevate his mood and
improve his "connection with the world."

Bryan eventually engages in a family meeting with Dr. Saunders, and his
parents express their love and concerns. His father peppers the doctor with
questions regarding the addictive properties of marijuana because he fears
that his son "will become a hard-core drug addict." His mother is more am-
bivalent regarding Bryan's use, and although she thinks it might be helpful for
his anxiety, she expresses concern as well. She cites "research" she has read
online indicating that marijuana can be used to treat ADHD. At the same time,
she worries that the drug might be causing her son's depression. Near the end
of the session, she describes her sister's schizophrenia and subsequent suicide,
as well as fears that Bryan's marijuana use could have the same consequence.

Dr. Saunders is puzzled by the complex questions that the Camellias
have raised, and she schedules a follow-up session. She wishes to give Bryan
and his family the most up-to-date, objective information about the risks and
any potential benefits of his marijuana use. She wonders: To what degree
does marijuana use lead to other drug problems? Does marijuana use help or
cause depression and anxiety? Does marijuana use help with ADHD?

Bryan, his parents, and Dr. Saunders all have unanswered questions about
the general behavioral health impacts of marijuana use, as well as its specific effects with regard to the most highly prevalent behavioral health conditions. Substance use disorders, mood disorders, anxiety disorders, and other behavioral
health disorders are affected by marijuana use, some in both positive and negative ways. Marijuana use can impact the risk of developing these conditions,
their course, and outcomes of the illnesses. In this chapter we present the available evidence on marijuana's impact on the risk, course, and outcomes of specific behavioral health conditions: substance use disorders, anxiety and mood
disorders, posttraumatic stress disorder (PTSD), ADHD, and sleep disturbances.
As shown in Table 5–1, for many of these conditions, research on associations
with marijuana use is limited, but it is possible to begin to answer some questions on the specific impact of marijuana use on these disorders. The complex
links between marijuana use and schizophrenia and related psychotic disorders
are reviewed in Chapter 6 ("Marijuana Use and Psychosis: From *Reefer Madness*
to Marijuana Use as a Component Cause").

Marijuana Use and Risk
for Substance Use Disorders

For much of the past century, scholars have sought to understand the patterns of progression of drug use. The earliest model from the 1930s was

TABLE 5–1. Marijuana use and associated behavioral health problems

Behavioral health problem	Strength of association[a]
Alcohol use	+++
Tobacco use	+++
Use of other illicit drugs	+
Bipolar disorder	++
Unipolar depression	+
Social anxiety	+++
Generalized anxiety	+
Panic disorder	+++
Posttraumatic stress disorder	+
Attention-deficit/hyperactivity disorder	+++
Sleep disturbances	+
Suicidality and violence	+

[a]Strength of association is indicated by +. These are merely associations and not necessarily causal relationships.

known as the *stepping stone theory,* which described a path from marijuana use to heroin addiction. Subsequent work in 1940s-era New York City challenged the inevitability of a progression from marijuana to opioid use (Cohen 1972). Later research established an alternative model: the *gateway hypothesis.* Unlike the stepping stone theory, the gateway hypothesis posits no causality, although it describes temporal patterns and progressions observed with drugs and alcohol.

The hypothesis that marijuana use is associated with the later use of other drugs has been long studied and is often cited (Fergusson et al. 2006; Yamaguchi and Kandel 1984b). More importantly, it has driven policy and legislation across the globe (Morral et al. 2002). The possibility of conflating association with causation complicates the search for truth and potentially misinforms important policy decisions. Here, we briefly examine the validity and utility of the gateway hypothesis and related models (Figure 5–1).

The gateway hypothesis comprises three related ideas: 1) that there is a developmental progression of drug use along a defined sequence of drugs, 2) that the use of certain drugs increases the risk of using other drugs, and 3) that the use of certain drugs causes the subsequent use of other drugs. Evidence for the first two ideas is vast, but the third causal model lacks robust scientific support (Kandel and Jessor 2002).

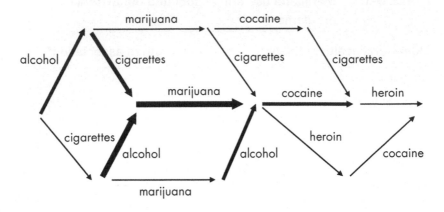

FIGURE 5–1. A model of the temporal progression of drug use.
Width of arrow conveys strength of association.
Source. Reprinted from Kandel DB: *Stages and Pathways of Drug Involvement: Examining the Gateway Hypothesis.* New York, Cambridge University Press, 2002. Copyright 2002, Cambridge University Press. Used with permission.

Marijuana and the Sequential Risk Model

The most widely supported developmental/temporal model for drug use begins with alcohol or tobacco and progresses to marijuana use and, finally, use of other illicit drugs such as cocaine or opioids (Fergusson et al. 2006; Lynskey et al. 2003b; Yamaguchi and Kandel 1984a). Kandel and colleagues (1992) found that alcohol use alone preceded marijuana use in men, and in women either alcohol or cigarette use was associated with later marijuana use. This is merely a temporal association whereby marijuana use typically follows legal drug use and precedes other illicit drug use. It is important to note that a causal relationship does not logically follow from this association. Observing a birth cohort of 1,265 New Zealand children over 21 years, Fergusson and Horwood (2000) found that the use of marijuana preceded other illicit drug use in 99% of cases. Conversely, only 37% of marijuana users progressed to other illicit drug use. The same group observed a clear dose-response association between marijuana use and other illicit drugs; for example, those subjects who used marijuana 50 or more times in a given year had a 140-fold increased rate of later illicit drug use (Fergusson and Horwood 2000).

These associations have been observed in many ethnic groups in different countries (e.g., the United States, France, Israel, Australia, Japan, Spain, and Scotland) over a 20-year period. Kandel (2002, p. 78) found associations between both earlier onset and frequency of marijuana use and later progression to other illicit drug use. This sequence can vary substantially among groups and social contexts. Some have considered that any association between marijuana use and other illicit drug use is entirely noncausal and merely subject to confounding factors such as drug availability, personality, adolescent developmental stages, lifestyle, or other nonobserved risk factors (Fergusson and Horwood 2000; Yamaguchi and Kandel 1984b).

To more adequately address the issue of causality, Fergusson et al. (2006) examined the aforementioned cohort of New Zealand children and controlled for multiple confounding factors. They found a strong association between increasing marijuana use and other illicit drug use, and this association varied with age. For instance, 15-year-olds who used marijuana weekly had a sixtyfold increase in risk for other illicit drug use; this same risk association fell substantially by age 25 to approximately fourfold. They also observed a dose-response relationship, in which increasing use of marijuana was associated with increased use and diversity of other illicit drug use. Ferguson and colleagues argued that the temporal sequence, dose-response relationship, strong association, and persistence of effects after controlling for confounding variables support a causal explanation for the association between marijuana use and other illicit drug use (Fergusson et al. 2006).

In addition, researchers have conducted twin studies to better understand how genetic and environmental factors may impact the association between marijuana use and drug use progression. Lynskey et al. (2003a) examined 311 twin pairs who were discordant for marijuana use. Those twins who used marijuana prior to age 17 had a 2.3- to 3.9-fold increased rate of other drug use compared with their abstinent twins. Their odds of developing alcohol dependence and other drug abuse or dependence were 1.6–6.0 times higher than the odds for their abstaining twins. These findings were consistent in both monozygotic and dizygotic twin pairs. Marijuana use prior to the age of 17 in both twins of a pair was significantly more common in monozygotic pairs relative to dizygotic pairs, suggesting an underlying genetic propensity for age at initiation of marijuana use. Although the study relied on retrospective self-report, the authors suggested that marijuana use may play a causal role in the development of further drug or alcohol use problems (Lynskey et al. 2003a). Additional evidence for a possible causal mechanism was elucidated by Agrawal and colleagues (2004). They analyzed data from 2,130 monozygotic and dizygotic twin pairs for associations between marijuana use and other illicit drug use and to determine whether one twin's marijuana use had an impact on the other twin's use of illicit drugs. They observed a strong association between marijuana use and abuse of or dependence on other illicit drugs. The associations within twin pairs were more robust for monozygotic twins relative to dizygotic ones, suggesting genetic underpinnings, although the researchers acknowledged that unrecognized environmental factors might also be at play (Agrawal et al. 2004).

Marijuana Use as a Gateway to Marijuana Use Disorders

Just as marijuana use may be a precedent, or "gateway," to further drug use, we should ask about the extent to which marijuana use is associated with later marijuana addiction or dependence. Work by Fergusson et al. (2003b), utilizing the same New Zealand birth cohort mentioned previously, revealed that a subjectively positive response to early marijuana use (prior to age 16) was associated with a twentyfold increase in rates of progression to marijuana dependence. Interestingly, negative experiences with marijuana were not associated with progression or lack of progression to dependence. Of the total sample, only 9% progressed to dependence by age 21, although 21.7% of those who used prior to age 16 progressed to marijuana dependence (Fergusson et al. 2003b).

Skepticism About a Causal Gateway Progression

Some have argued that the evidence supporting a gateway progression is spurious and subject to confounding variables such as cultural attitudes, drug availability, or other unobserved common causes that underlie the risk for developing addiction. Relevant work from Degenhardt et al. (2010) assessed whether the gateway hypothesis holds true in an array of diverse countries. Using the World Health Organization's World Mental Health Surveys from 17 developing and developed countries, the authors found that the gateway hypothesis was not consistently supported in all countries. In most instances, drugs used earlier in the sequence predicted drug use later in the sequence. However, the strength of these associations varied among countries. Rather than being strictly causal, the associations in drug use progression were related to background prevalence of use of individual drugs. For instance, in Japan, where exposure and access to marijuana were less common, the authors did not observe an associated reduction in levels of other illicit drug use as might be expected from a strictly causal model (Degenhardt et al. 2010).

Furthering this line of work, Morral et al. (2002) examined whether the gateway progression could be wholly explained by a common factor of propensity for drug use. Utilizing U.S. household surveys of drug use between 1982 and 1994, the authors built a model of drug use progression without assuming a causal gateway phenomenon. Associations, drug use ordering, and dose responses from this common factor model reproduced those observed in prior studies. Although these findings did not rule out the possibility of a gateway causal mechanism, they supported the theory that a common factor, such as propensity for drug use, could explain the observed gateway phenomenon (Morral et al. 2002).

Marijuana and the Priming Effect

Complementing the population-based studies are animal models that support a cannabinoid-mediated mechanism for "priming" the brain for addiction. Research suggests that a periadolescent, developing brain may be uniquely sensitive when exposed to cannabinoids. Such exposure can induce a long-lasting cross-tolerance to other drugs (opioids, cocaine, amphetamine) in the dopaminergic reward centers of the adolescent rat brain (Panlilio et al. 2013; Pistis et al. 2004).

Clinical Relevance

From a clinical perspective, it is important to consider whether marijuana use may increase the risk for future drug use problems. The extant body of research shows that marijuana use, particularly at a young age or greater frequency, is associated with a progression to other illicit drugs. However, such an association is not absolute, and it likely is multidetermined with other genetic, environmental, and social factors. Nonetheless, clinicians should be aware of such associations and counsel patients and those involved in their care regarding these patterns. Such education may help mitigate the risk of progression to drug use disorders.

Marijuana Use and Anxiety and Mood Disorders

The comorbidity between marijuana use and mood and anxiety disorders has been well documented in the literature across many diverse populations (Grant et al. 2004; Saban et al. 2014; Wu et al. 2013). Although there is no debate that these behavioral health conditions often co-occur, considerable debate exists on the causal relationships between marijuana use and mood and anxiety disorders. The debate is quite nuanced and ranges from theories of marijuana use as a form of self-medication and coping with anxiety and depression to theories that use of marijuana, particularly earlier in adolescence, results in greater risk of anxiety and depression in adulthood. Similarly, research has examined marijuana and specific cannabinoids as potentially effective pharmaceutical interventions for the treatment of depression and anxiety. In the United States, mood disorders, including major depressive disorder and bipolar disorder, and anxiety disorders, including social anxiety disorder, panic disorder, and generalized anxiety disorder (GAD), are some of the most highly prevalent psychiatric disorders across all age groups. Marijuana is the most commonly used illicit drug. Thus, the comorbid associations between these behavioral health conditions, including risk, course, and outcomes, are particularly relevant and of substantial clinical interest.

One major source of debate in research on marijuana use and causality relates to the wide range of responses to marijuana use that individuals can experience. On one end of the spectrum, individuals using marijuana can experience positive responses, including relaxation, euphoria, and heightened perception. On the other end of the spectrum, those using marijuana can experience dysphoria, anxiety, and unpleasant perceptual distortions (Pacher et al. 2006). This varied response relates to the fact that there can be either enhancement or blockade of endocannabinoid neurotransmission, resulting in anxiolytic or anxiogenic effects (Witkin et al. 2005).

According to the National Comorbidity Survey, approximately 90% of respondents with a diagnosis of cannabis dependence had a lifetime prevalence of any mental disorder, compared with 55% of respondents without cannabis dependence (Agosti et al. 2002). Again, with large epidemiological, cross-sectional studies, causality is often unclear. Even retrospectively establishing whether anxiety and depressive symptoms precede marijuana use or vice versa is difficult. Whereas some studies have found that the onset of mood and anxiety symptoms precedes marijuana use and dependence (Agosti et al. 2002; Wittchen et al. 2007), others have found that marijuana use leads to increased risk of mood disorders (depression and, more strongly, bipolar disorder) without increasing the risk of anxiety disorders (van Laar et al. 2007). Another study, involving Australian youth and young adults, found a threefold increase in risk of depression and anxiety symptoms in adulthood among early and more frequent young marijuana users (Hayatbakhsh et al. 2007).

Marijuana Use and Anxiety Disorders

Associations between various anxiety disorders and marijuana use have been studied in a number of settings. In a meta-analysis of anxiety and marijuana use and marijuana use disorders, small positive associations were found between anxiety and marijuana use (odds ratio [OR] = 1.24) and cannabis use disorders (OR = 1.68) and between comorbid anxiety and depression and marijuana use (OR = 1.68) (Kedzior and Laeber 2014). Other studies have found either no association or little association between marijuana use and anxiety disorders (Tournier et al. 2003). The precise mechanisms of the relationship between anxiety disorders and marijuana use remain unclear (Crippa et al. 2009).

Much research has evaluated the relationship between social anxiety disorder and marijuana use. A causal association may exist between a diagnosis of social anxiety disorder and use of marijuana. Because many people self-medicate with alcohol to reduce anxiety in social situations, research has found a possible similar phenomenon in some adolescents, who may smoke marijuana to decrease anxiety in specific social settings (Comeau et al. 2001). In fact, social anxiety disorder is an identified risk factor for cannabis dependence and has been associated with 6.5 times greater odds of developing cannabis dependence (Buckner et al. 2007, 2008). Furthermore, in the National Epidemiologic Survey on Alcohol and Related Conditions (NESARC), social anxiety disorder was diagnosed prior to the onset of cannabis use disorders for most individuals with comorbid cannabis use disorders and social anxiety disorder, and this combination of conditions was more difficult to treat than either condition alone (Buckner et al. 2012).

Less research exists on the association between GAD and marijuana use disorders, and the results are inconsistent (Wittchen et al. 2007). GAD and marijuana use disorders are common comorbid conditions (Grant et al. 2004), and many studies have found evidence to support that marijuana is a self-medication or coping mechanism for anxiety symptoms (Bonn-Miller et al. 2008; Zvolensky et al. 2007). Additional research is needed to better understand the nature of the relationship between GAD and marijuana use.

The anxiety disorder most consistently associated with marijuana use is panic disorder. The consistency of this association may be related to panic attacks at times being an acute adverse experience associated with marijuana use (Crippa et al. 2009; Thomas 1996; Wittchen et al. 2007). A lifetime history of marijuana use is associated with increased risk of a panic attack or a diagnosis of panic disorder, and more frequent marijuana use is associated with panic attacks (Zvolensky et al. 2006, 2010). One small study found an association between agoraphobia and marijuana use in a sample of college students (Tournier et al. 2003).

Marijuana Use and Mood Disorders

Similar to anxiety disorders, mood disorders have also been inconsistently associated with marijuana use. Large national epidemiological surveys have found some emerging patterns in this association. The 1980 Baltimore Epidemiologic Catchment Area study found that individuals who used marijuana at baseline had four times greater rates of depressive symptoms (especially suicidal ideation and anhedonia) than those who did not use marijuana (Bovasso 2001). The National Comorbidity Survey found an association between the number of occasions of marijuana use and a first major depressive episode (Chen et al. 2002). In the National Longitudinal

Survey of Youth, children were surveyed in 1979 and again as adults in 1994. Among the adults surveyed, rates of depression were 1.4 times higher among past-year marijuana users when compared with those not using marijuana. However, adjustment for differences in risk factors of marijuana use and depression led to virtual elimination of these findings (Harder et al. 2006). Other studies have also shown associations that do not hold after adjustment; for example, in a sample of Australian adults, marijuana use was associated with increasing rates of anxiety and mood disorders until the study authors controlled for demographics, neuroticism, and other drug use (Degenhardt et al. 2001).

There are ongoing challenges in establishing causality between marijuana use and mood disorders. In one study using NESARC data, when the presence of mood disorders was controlled for at baseline, marijuana use was not associated with an increase in depression, but *regular* use (weekly to almost daily) was associated with bipolar disorder (OR=2.47), although daily use was not. This study did not find an association between depression and marijuana use, and the link between bipolar disorder and marijuana use requires further study (Feingold et al. 2014).

Clinical Relevance

Whether or not marijuana use is an effective method of self-medication for anxiety disorders and mood disorders remains unclear. The *coping hypothesis,* which suggests that many people use marijuana to cope with symptoms of anxiety and depression, has been examined in the context of disasters; for example, rates of marijuana use increased after the September 11, 2001 terrorist attacks (Vlahov et al. 2004). However, among Manhattan residents, depression prevalence was greater for individuals who increased marijuana use than for those who did not (22.3% vs. 9.4%) (Vlahov et al. 2002).

There is a well-described withdrawal syndrome associated with marijuana use cessation (Hasin et al. 2008). Some users note increased irritability and anxiety (Budney et al. 2004), and many studies have examined various methods to treat anxiety as part of effective cannabis dependence treatment (Haney et al. 2003, 2004). Regarding individuals with bipolar disorder, the European Mania in Bipolar Longitudinal Evaluation of Medication (EMBLEM) study found that patients who stopped using marijuana had similar outcomes to those who had never used it (in terms of recurrence, remission, recovery, and relapse of manic/mixed episodes), compared with those who continued to use (Zorrilla et al. 2015).

A dual theme emerges with regard to marijuana use and anxiety disorders. There is ample evidence to support the association between increased rates of specific anxiety disorders among individuals who use marijuana, particularly in younger individuals and those who begin using marijuana at an earlier age. However, there is also some evidence that supports the consideration of marijuana—and potentially specific compounds interacting with cannabinoid type 1 (CB_1) receptors—as possible future treatment options for various anxiety disorders, particularly social anxiety disorder (Bergamaschi et al. 2011; Hill and Gorzalka 2009). More rigorous and controlled research is needed.

Marijuana Use and Risk, Course, and Outcomes of Other Psychiatric Disorders

Posttraumatic Stress Disorder

It is well established that individuals with PTSD have increased rates of substance use disorders, particularly alcohol abuse or dependence (Kessler et al. 1995). It is possible that substance use predisposes persons to the development of traumatic exposures and PTSD. Conversely, the model that PTSD precedes substance use disorders has gained traction (Jacobsen et al. 2001).

Although there is no evidence that marijuana use is a risk factor for developing PTSD, there is evidence that the development of PTSD predisposes individuals to use of alcohol and other substances. Breslau et al. (2003) found that PTSD, as opposed to trauma alone, was associated with an increased risk of drug use in a cohort of young adult civilians. However, these findings did not distinguish marijuana from the other drugs included in the study. Another group found that PTSD preceded the abuse of psychoactive prescribed drugs, although it did not lead to the abuse of illicit drugs such as cocaine and marijuana (Chilcoat and Breslau 1998).

A study of approximately 3,000 St. Louis residents in the 1980s found that marijuana use was protective against the development of PTSD, although it was associated with a slightly higher rate of traumatic events (Cottler et al. 1992). This finding requires further exploration.

Attention-Deficit/Hyperactivity Disorder

Some evidence indicates that ADHD in childhood is a risk factor for developing substance misuse (particularly marijuana use) in adulthood; however, there is less clear evidence on the impact of marijuana use on ADHD course and outcomes (Dunne et al. 2014; Sibley et al. 2014; Vitulano et al. 2014). Specific subtypes of ADHD may be more closely related to the risk of marijuana use, with the inattention type having a greater association with severity of use and with hyperactivity-impulsivity being associated with earlier age at initiation of marijuana use (Bidwell et al. 2014). Although very little research exists on outcomes of ADHD associated with marijuana use, one recent study found poorer ADHD outcomes (i.e., worsening inattention, less improvement of hyperactivity and impulsivity) among adolescents with early marijuana use (Howard et al. 2015).

Sleep Disturbances

The relationship between marijuana use and sleep is two-pronged in that both intoxication and withdrawal states must be considered. Marijuana use is associated with reduced rapid eye movement sleep, shorter sleep-onset latency, and increased stage 4 sleep (Schierenbeck et al. 2008). Sedative effects have been observed to persist into the following day (Schierenbeck et al. 2008). Insomnia and "strange dreams" are the most common sleep effects associated with marijuana withdrawal (Schierenbeck et al. 2008). Among heavy marijuana users, sleep problems were identified at higher rates after discontinuation of marijuana use. It would also appear that sleep problems in early childhood (ages 3–5) can predict use of marijuana and alcohol in adolescence and early adulthood (Wong et al. 2004).

Marijuana Use and Social Determinants of Mental Health

The social determinants of mental health—those social factors that affect mental health (i.e., where and under what circumstances individuals grow, work, live, play, and age)—have direct impacts on mental health and substance use disorders, including marijuana use disorders, mood disorders, and anxiety disorders. Furthermore, it is possible that marijuana use has impacts on risk, course, and outcomes of mental illnesses by affecting social determinants of mental health (e.g., by leading to poorer educational outcomes and thus lower employment and decreased income potential). There is an association between early marijuana use and mental health problems in adulthood, but these associations may be mediated by education; employment status; marital status; and use of other drugs, especially alcohol and tobacco (Green and Ritter 2000). Unfortunately, marijuana (especially early use) is associated with poor educational achievement and high school dropout (Fergusson et al. 2003a; Lynskey and Hall 2000; Lynskey et al. 2003a). The association between marijuana use and poor educational outcomes may be the result of interactions between various social determinants of mental health (e.g., poverty, adverse early childhood experiences, social exclusion), or other social and environmental risk factors (Verweij et al. 2013).

Marijuana Use and Risk for Violence and Suicide

Alcohol is the prototypical drug associated with an increased risk of violence and suicide. The evidence linking marijuana to violence is drastically less robust. Although routine or "regular" marijuana dosages for a given user are not associated with a risk of violence, atypical or high doses may bring a slight, although perhaps not statistically significant, increase in risk (Haggård-Grann et al. 2006). Using data from a large birth cohort from Dunedin, New Zealand, Arseneault et al. (2002) observed an increased risk of violence in those with alcohol dependence, marijuana dependence, or schizophrenia spectrum illnesses. However, the association between increased risk of violence and marijuana dependence may be due to the illicit nature of the marijuana drug market.

The relationship between marijuana use and suicide is even more muddled. A longitudinal study of more than 50,000 Swedish men older than 33 years found a positive association between ever using marijuana and death by suicide (OR=1.62). However, this relationship did not persist when considering confounding factors such as socioeconomic status, age, alcohol and tobacco use, and psychiatric diagnoses (Price et al. 2009). To further complicate the picture, another study longitudinally followed 2,033 Norwegian adolescents older than 13 years and attempted to control for a large group of potential confounding variables. The authors observed a positive relationship between any marijuana use and suicidal thinking (OR=2.4–2.7). Heavier use was associated with an increased risk of suicide attempts (OR=2.8) (Pedersen 2008).

Key Points

- Marijuana use is one of many factors that have impacts on mental health, although its independent effects are difficult to disentangle from confounding biological, psychological, and social factors.
- Marijuana use does not inexorably lead to, or cause, other substance use disorders, although it often begins after initiation of alcohol and tobacco use. Although a majority of people who use cocaine or opioids used marijuana previously, a relatively small percentage of those who use marijuana progress to other illicit drug use. Those who use marijuana more heavily, or who begin their use earlier in life, may be particularly at risk for further drug use problems.
- Although marijuana use does not solely cause or cure mental health problems, it has been associated with some of them. Marijuana use is most strongly associated with panic disorder, attention-deficit/

hyperactivity disorder, and social anxiety. Use during early adolescence may confer an increased risk of anxiety and depression in adulthood.

- Although marijuana use may be a risk factor for violence and suicide, it does not, in itself, cause either.

References

Agosti V, Nunes E, Levin F: Rates of psychiatric comorbidity among U.S. residents with lifetime cannabis dependence. Am J Drug Alcohol Abuse 28(4):643–652, 2002 12492261

Agrawal A, Neale MC, Prescott CA, et al: A twin study of early cannabis use and subsequent use and abuse/dependence of other illicit drugs. Psychol Med 34(7):1227–1237, 2004 15697049

Arseneault L, Moffit TE, Caspi A, et al: The targets of violence committed by young offenders with alcohol dependence, marijuana dependence and schizophrenia-spectrum disorders: findings from a birth cohort. Crim Behav Ment Health 12(2):155–168, 2002 12459816

Bergamaschi MM, Queiroz RHC, Chagas MHN, et al: Cannabidiol reduces the anxiety induced by simulated public speaking in treatment-naïve social phobia patients. Neuropsychopharmacology 36(6):1219–1226, 2011 21307846

Bidwell LC, Henry EA, Willcutt EG, et al: Childhood and current ADHD symptom dimensions are associated with more severe cannabis outcomes in college students. Drug Alcohol Depend 135:88–94, 2014 24332802

Bonn-Miller MO, Zvolensky MJ, Bernstein A, et al: Marijuana coping motives interact with marijuana use frequency to predict anxious arousal, panic related catastrophic thinking, and worry among current marijuana users. Depress Anxiety 25(10):862–873, 2008 17849459

Bovasso GB: Cannabis abuse as a risk factor for depressive symptoms. Am J Psychiatry 158(12):2033–2037, 2001 11729021

Breslau N, Davis GC, Schultz LR: Posttraumatic stress disorder and the incidence of nicotine, alcohol, and other drug disorders in persons who have experienced trauma. Arch Gen Psychiatry 60(3):289–294, 2003 12622662

Buckner JD, Bonn-Miller MO, Zvolensky MJ, et al: Marijuana use motives and social anxiety among marijuana-using young adults. Addict Behav 32(10):2238–2252, 2007 17478056

Buckner JD, Schmidt NB, Lang AR, et al: Specificity of social anxiety disorder as a risk factor for alcohol and cannabis dependence. J Psychiatr Res 42(3):230–239, 2008 17320907

Buckner JD, Heimberg RG, Schneier FR, et al: The relationship between cannabis use disorders and social anxiety disorder in the National Epidemiological Study of Alcohol and Related Conditions (NESARC). Drug Alcohol Depend 124(1–2):128–134, 2012 22266089

Budney AJ, Hughes JR, Moore BA, et al: Review of the validity and significance of cannabis withdrawal syndrome. Am J Psychiatry 161(11):1967–1977, 2004 15514394

Chen CY, Wagner FA, Anthony JC: Marijuana use and the risk of major depressive episode: epidemiological evidence from the United States National Comorbidity Survey. Soc Psychiatry Psychiatr Epidemiol 37(5):199–206, 2002 12107710

Chilcoat HD, Breslau N: Posttraumatic stress disorder and drug disorders: testing causal pathways. Arch Gen Psychiatry 55(10):913–917, 1998 9783562

Cohen H: Multiple drug use considered in the light of the stepping-stone hypothesis. Int J Addict 7(1):27–55, 1972 5043838

Comeau N, Stewart SH, Loba P: The relations of trait anxiety, anxiety sensitivity, and sensation seeking to adolescents' motivations for alcohol, cigarette, and marijuana use. Addict Behav 26(6):803–825, 2001 11768546

Cottler LB, Compton WM III, Mager D, et al: Posttraumatic stress disorder among substance users from the general population. Am J Psychiatry 149(5):664–670, 1992 1575258

Crippa JA, Zuardi AW, Martín-Santos R, et al: Cannabis and anxiety: a critical review of the evidence. Hum Psychopharmacol 24(7):515–523, 2009 19693792

Degenhardt L, Hall W, Lynskey M: Alcohol, cannabis and tobacco use among Australians: a comparison of their associations with other drug use and use disorders, affective and anxiety disorders, and psychosis. Addiction 96(11):1603–1614, 2001 11784457

Degenhardt L, Dierker L, Chiu WT, et al: Evaluating the drug use "gateway" theory using cross-national data: consistency and associations of the order of initiation of drug use among participants in the WHO World Mental Health Surveys. Drug Alcohol Depend 108(1–2):84–97, 2010 20060657

Dunne EM, Hearn LE, Rose JJ, et al: ADHD as a risk factor for early onset and heightened adult problem severity of illicit substance use: an accelerated gateway model. Addict Behav 39(12):1755–1758, 2014 25123341

Feingold D, Weiser M, Rehm J, et al: The association between cannabis use and mood disorders: a longitudinal study. J Affect Disord 172C:211–218, 2014 25451420

Fergusson DM, Horwood LJ: Does cannabis use encourage other forms of illicit drug use? Addiction 95(4):505–520, 2000 10829327

Fergusson DM, Horwood LJ, Beautrais AL: Cannabis and educational achievement. Addiction 98(12):1681–1692, 2003a 14651500

Fergusson DM, Horwood LJ, Lynskey MT, et al: Early reactions to cannabis predict later dependence. Arch Gen Psychiatry 60(10):1033–1039, 2003b 14557149

Fergusson DM, Boden JM, Horwood LJ: Cannabis use and other illicit drug use: testing the cannabis gateway hypothesis. Addiction 101(4):556–569, 2006 16548935

Grant BF, Stinson FS, Dawson DA, et al: Prevalence and co-occurrence of substance use disorders and independent mood and anxiety disorders: results from the National Epidemiologic Survey on Alcohol and Related Conditions. Arch Gen Psychiatry 61(8):807–816, 2004 15289279

Green BE, Ritter C: Marijuana use and depression. J Health Soc Behav 41(1):40–49, 2000 10750321

Haggård-Grann U, Hallqvist J, Långström N, et al: The role of alcohol and drugs in triggering criminal violence: a case-crossover study. Addiction 101(1):100–108, 2006 16393196

Haney M, Hart CL, Ward AS, et al: Nefazodone decreases anxiety during marijuana withdrawal in humans. Psychopharmacology (Berl) 165(2):157–165, 2003 12439626

Haney M, Hart CL, Vosburg SK, et al: Marijuana withdrawal in humans: effects of oral THC or divalproex. Neuropsychopharmacology 29(1):158–170, 2004 14560320

Harder VS, Morral AR, Arkes J: Marijuana use and depression among adults: testing for causal associations. Addiction 101(10):1463–1472, 2006 16968348

Hasin DS, Keyes KM, Alderson D, et al: Cannabis withdrawal in the United States: results from NESARC. J Clin Psychiatry 69(9):1354–1363, 2008 19012815

Hayatbakhsh MR, Najman JM, Jamrozik K, et al: Cannabis and anxiety and depression in young adults: a large prospective study. J Am Acad Child Adolesc Psychiatry 46(3):408–417, 2007 17314727

Hill MN, Gorzalka BB: The endocannabinoid system and the treatment of mood and anxiety disorders. CNS Neurol Disord Drug Targets 8(6):451–458, 2009 19839936

Howard AL, Molina BSG, Swanson JM, et al: Developmental progression to early adult binge drinking and marijuana use from worsening versus stable trajectories of adolescent attention deficit/hyperactivity disorder and delinquency. Addiction 110(5):784–795, 2015 25664657

Jacobsen LK, Southwick SM, Kosten TR: Substance use disorders in patients with posttraumatic stress disorder: a review of the literature. Am J Psychiatry 158(8):1184–1190, 2001 11481147

Kandel DB (ed): Stages and Pathways of Drug Involvement: Examining the Gateway Hypothesis. New York, Cambridge University Press, 2002

Kandel DB, Jessor R: The gateway hypothesis revisited, in Stages and Pathways of Drug Involvement: Examining the Gateway Hypothesis. Edited by Kandel DB. New York, Cambridge University Press, 2002, pp 365–372

Kandel DB, Yamaguchi K, Chen K: Stages of progression in drug involvement from adolescence to adulthood: further evidence for the gateway theory. J Stud Alcohol 53(5):447–457, 1992 1405637

Kedzior KK, Laeber LT: A positive association between anxiety disorders and cannabis use or cannabis use disorders in the general population—a meta-analysis of 31 studies. BMC Psychiatry 14:136, 2014 24884989

Kessler RC, Sonnega A, Bromet E, et al: Posttraumatic stress disorder in the National Comorbidity Survey. Arch Gen Psychiatry 52(12):1048–1060, 1995 7492257

Lynskey M, Hall W: The effects of adolescent cannabis use on educational attainment: a review. Addiction 95(11):1621–1630, 2000 11219366

Lynskey MT, Coffey C, Degenhardt L, et al: A longitudinal study of the effects of adolescent cannabis use on high school completion. Addiction 98(5):685–692, 2003a 12751986

Lynskey MT, Heath AC, Bucholz KK, et al: Escalation of drug use in early onset cannabis users vs co-twin controls. JAMA 289(4):427–433, 2003b 12533121

Morral AR, McCaffrey DF, Paddock SM: Reassessing the marijuana gateway effect. Addiction 97(12):1493–1504, 2002 12472629

Pacher P, Bátkai S, Kunos G: The endocannabinoid system as an emerging target of pharmacotherapy. Pharmacol Rev 58(3):389–462, 2006 16968947

Panlilio LV, Zanettini C, Barnes C, et al: Prior exposure to THC increases the addictive effects of nicotine in rats. Neuropsychopharmacology 38(7):1198–1208, 2013 23314220

Pedersen W: Does cannabis use lead to depression and suicidal behaviours? A population-based longitudinal study. Acta Psychiatr Scand 118(5):395–403, 2008 18798834

Pistis M, Perra S, Pillolla G, et al: Adolescent exposure to cannabinoids induces long-lasting changes in the response to drugs of abuse of rat midbrain dopamine neurons. Biol Psychiatry 56(2):86–94, 2004 15231440

Price C, Hemmingsson T, Lewis G, et al: Cannabis and suicide: longitudinal study. Br J Psychiatry 195(6):492–497, 2009 19949196

Saban A, Flisher AJ, Grimsrud A, et al: The association between substance use and common mental disorders in young adults: results from the South African Stress and Health (SASH) Survey. Pan Afr Med J 17 (suppl 1):11, 2014 24624244

Schierenbeck T, Riemann D, Berger M, et al: Effect of illicit recreational drugs upon sleep: cocaine, ecstasy and marijuana. Sleep Med Rev 12(5):381–389, 2008 18313952

Sibley MH, Pelham WE, Molina BSG, et al: The role of early childhood ADHD and subsequent CD in the initiation and escalation of adolescent cigarette, alcohol, and marijuana use. J Abnorm Psychol 123(2):362–374, 2014 24886010

Thomas H: A community survey of adverse effects of cannabis use. Drug Alcohol Depend 42(3):201–207, 1996 8912803

Tournier M, Sorbara F, Gindre C, et al: Cannabis use and anxiety in daily life: a naturalistic investigation in a non-clinical population. Psychiatry Res 118(1):1–8, 2003 12759155

van Laar M, van Dorsselaer S, Monshouwer K, et al: Does cannabis use predict the first incidence of mood and anxiety disorders in the adult population? Addiction 102(8):1251–1260, 2007 17624975

Verweij KJH, Huizink AC, Agrawal A, et al: Is the relationship between early onset cannabis use and educational attainment causal or due to common liability? Drug Alcohol Depend 133(2):580–586, 2013 23972999

Vitulano ML, Fite PJ, Hopko DR, et al: Evaluation of underlying mechanisms in the link between childhood ADHD symptoms and risk for early initiation of substance use. Psychol Addict Behav 28(3):816–827, 2014 25222174

Vlahov D, Galea S, Resnick H, et al: Increased use of cigarettes, alcohol, and marijuana among Manhattan, New York, residents after the September 11th terrorist attacks. Am J Epidemiol 155(11):988–996, 2002 12034577

Vlahov D, Galea S, Ahern J, et al: Consumption of cigarettes, alcohol, and marijuana among New York City residents six months after the September 11 terrorist attacks. Am J Drug Alcohol Abuse 30(2):385–407, 2004 15230082

Witkin JM, Tzavara ET, Nomikos GG: A role for cannabinoid CB1 receptors in mood and anxiety disorders. Behav Pharmacol 16(5–6):315–331, 2005 16148437

Wittchen HU, Fröhlich C, Behrendt S, et al: Cannabis use and cannabis use disorders and their relationship to mental disorders: a 10-year prospective-longitudinal community study in adolescents. Drug Alcohol Depend 88 (suppl 1):S60–S70, 2007 17257779

Wong MM, Brower KJ, Fitzgerald HE, et al: Sleep problems in early childhood and early onset of alcohol and other drug use in adolescence. Alcohol Clin Exp Res 28(4):578–587, 2004 15100609

Wu LT, Blazer DG, Gersing KR, et al: Comorbid substance use disorders with other Axis I and II mental disorders among treatment-seeking Asian Americans, Native Hawaiians/Pacific Islanders, and mixed-race people. J Psychiatr Res 47(12):1940–1948, 2013 24060266

Yamaguchi K, Kandel DB: Patterns of drug use from adolescence to young adulthood, II: sequences of progression. Am J Public Health 74(7):668–672, 1984a 6742252

Yamaguchi K, Kandel DB: Patterns of drug use from adolescence to young adulthood, III: predictors of progression. Am J Public Health 74(7):673–681, 1984b 6742253

Zorrilla I, Aguado J, Haro JM, et al: Cannabis and bipolar disorder: does quitting cannabis use during manic/mixed episode improve clinical/functional outcomes? Acta Psychiatr Scand 131(2):100–110, 2015 25430820

Zvolensky MJ, Bernstein A, Sachs-Ericsson N, et al: Lifetime associations between cannabis use, abuse, and dependence and panic attacks in a representative sample. J Psychiatr Res 40(6):477–486, 2006 16271364

Zvolensky MJ, Vujanovic AA, Bernstein A, et al: Marijuana use motives: a confirmatory test and evaluation among young adult marijuana users. Addict Behav 32(12):3122–3130, 2007 17602842

Zvolensky MJ, Cougle JR, Johnson KA, et al: Marijuana use and panic psychopathology among a representative sample of adults. Exp Clin Psychopharmacol 18(2):129–134, 2010 20384424

CHAPTER 6

Marijuana Use and Psychosis

From *Reefer Madness* to Marijuana Use as a Component Cause

Claire Ramsay Wan, M.P.H.
Michael T. Compton, M.D., M.P.H.

Clinical Vignette: Andrew's Psychotic Disorder in the Context of Marijuana Use

Maggie Harlan is a physician assistant employed in a private pediatric practice at a suburban wellness center. She provides general pediatric care to children and adolescents and refers her patients as needed to psychiatry, physical therapy, and nutrition services provided at the same location. Her next appointment is with Andrew Farrel, a 17-year-old whom she has known for 6 years.

Nancy Farrel brought her son Andrew in today with a concern that "something is wrong" with him. His grades from last semester were terrible, he was fired from his summer job for absenteeism, and he "became obsessed" with playing video games at night. His parents sent him to a month-long youth retreat in another state but were asked to pick him up after 3 weeks because he was not participating in activities or bathing regularly and was seen talking to himself. Nancy picked him up and brought him straight to the pediatric practice.

After his mother leaves the room, Andrew reluctantly admits that he has been smoking marijuana heavily for several years and has lost any interest in doing other activities, except for playing video games. He reports smoking almost daily until he went to the youth retreat, where he did not have access to the drug. When asked about his obsession with video games, he quietly asserts that the characters started talking to him about 5 weeks ago while he was high. He says that they began nagging him about "completing his mission" whenever he tried to sleep and that they followed him to the youth retreat and became angry with him. When asked about the mission, he talks about how each game level represents a place on Earth that is under attack and says that he must provide defense to prevent "bad things" from happening to the people who live on the level with us all.

Maggie empathizes with Andrew's distress and facilitates a difficult conversation between Andrew and Nancy about some of his experiences and his marijuana use. She also consults a psychiatrist down the hall, who agrees to meet Andrew for further evaluation and treatment planning. Nancy asks many questions about her son's condition and the role that marijuana played in the development of his symptoms. Some of the questions Nancy asks include the following: What is Andrew's diagnosis? Is it common to see marijuana use accompanied by delusions such as this? Did the marijuana cause Andrew's illness, or did it make his symptoms worse? If Andrew stops smoking marijuana, will he get better?

Co-occurrence of Marijuana Use and Psychosis

Differentiating Primary and Secondary Psychotic Disorders

Psychosis is defined as a condition in which the affected individual loses touch with external reality. This can be manifested by delusions, hallucinations, or disorganized thoughts or grossly disorganized behavior. *Delusions* are fixed, false beliefs that continue to be held despite evidence to the contrary. The content of delusions can vary widely and can include persecutory beliefs (e.g., that others are harassing, following, watching, or plotting against the affected person), grandiose beliefs (e.g., that the affected individual is famous or has extraordinary abilities), or referential beliefs (e.g., that others are talking about the affected person or that environmental factors are directed toward the affected person). Delusions must be differentiated from cultural norms in the individual's community.

Hallucinations are sensory perceptions in absence of external stimuli. The most common sensory modality in which hallucinations manifest is auditory (such as hearing voices or noises), but visual, olfactory, tactile, and gustatory hallucinations can occur. Hallucinations are usually perceived clearly, are not under voluntary control, and occur while the affected individual is fully awake. Disorganized thoughts are typically inferred from the affected individual's speech patterns and must be involuntary and severe to constitute psychosis. Examples of disorganized speech include *derailment* or *loose associations,* in which the individual unexpectedly changes from one topic to another; *tangentiality,* meaning that answers to questions are oblique or gradually become unrelated to the original question; and *word salad,* in which words are spoken without forming sentences or clear thoughts.

Psychosis may occur independently or in the context of a variety of psychiatric and medical illnesses, including depression, mania, delirium, dementia, vitamin deficiency, brain lesion, and toxicity. DSM-5 (American Psychiatric Association 2013) states that secondary causes of psychosis should be ruled out before a diagnosis of a primary psychotic disorder is made. Thus, the typical workup for new-onset psychosis should include investigations for potential toxicity, infection, anatomic central nervous system lesion, thyroid abnormality, and vitamin B_{12} deficiency, among others, as a cause of the patient's symptoms. Additionally, psychotic symptoms may occur in the context of an affective disorder such as bipolar disorder or major depressive disorder. If the patient has a major depressive disorder or history of manic episodes, the clinician should first consider a diagnosis of an affective disorder with psychotic features, then a diagnosis of schizoaffective disorder, before considering a diagnosis of a primary psychotic disorder.

Substances that can elicit psychotic symptoms during either intoxication or withdrawal are listed in Table 6–1 (American Psychiatric Association 2013). To meet the diagnostic criteria outlined in DSM-5, substance-induced psychotic disorder (SIPD) must be characterized by prominent hallucinations or delusions. The affected individual may also present with negative symptoms and disorganized thoughts or behaviors. The hallucinations or delusions must be judged to be attributable to the physiological effects of the substance and must cause distress for the patient or his or her family or friends. Of note, hallucinations that are recognized as unreal by the patient do not qualify for SIPD and are instead classified as perceptual abnormalities secondary to substance use. SIPD typically emerges shortly after the initial use of or withdrawal from the substance in question, but symptoms may persist long term during continued use and for several weeks after the substance use is discontinued.

Once secondary causes of psychosis have been ruled out, the clinician should consider a diagnosis of a primary psychotic, or *schizophrenia spectrum,* disorder. Diagnostic criteria for some of these disorders, which include presence of one or more symptoms over a specified duration of time, are

TABLE 6–1.   Substances of abuse that can induce psychosis

Recreational drugs that can provoke psychotic symptoms during intoxication	Recreational drugs that can provoke psychotic symptoms during withdrawal
Alcohol	Alcohol
Anxiolytics	Anxiolytics
Hallucinogens (including phencyclidine)	Hypnotics
Hypnotics	Sedatives
Inhalants	
Marijuana	
Sedatives	
Stimulants (e.g., cocaine)	

Source.   American Psychiatric Association 2013.

shown in Boxes 6–1 through 6–4. In addition to delusions, hallucinations, and disorganized thoughts, the clinician should consider the presence or absence of disorganized behaviors and negative symptoms when forming a diagnosis. Laboratory tests to confirm psychotic disorder diagnoses do not yet exist, and imaging studies are not currently of clinical utility for primary psychotic disorder diagnosis (although neuroimaging is often included in the initial workup to rule out overt central nervous system pathology). The peak age at onset is in the 20s, but symptoms may develop as early as childhood and as late as mid-adulthood (and, rarely, in late adulthood). Men typically have an earlier age at onset (late adolescence to mid-20s), whereas women typically present later in their 20s and have a second, albeit smaller, peak of onset in mid-adulthood.

Box 6–1.   DSM-5 Diagnostic Criteria for Brief Psychotic Disorder

A. Presence of one (or more) of the following symptoms. At least one of these must be (1), (2), or (3):

1. Delusions.
2. Hallucinations.
3. Disorganized speech (e.g., frequent derailment or incoherence).
4. Grossly disorganized or catatonic behavior.

Note: Do not include a symptom if it is a culturally sanctioned response.

B. Duration of an episode of the disturbance is at least 1 day but less than 1 month, with eventual full return to premorbid level of functioning.

C. The disturbance is not better explained by major depressive or bipolar disorder with psychotic features or another psychotic disorder such as schizophrenia or catatonia, and is not attributable to the physiological effects of a substance (e.g., a drug of abuse, a medication) or another medical condition.

Specify if:

With marked stressor(s) (brief reactive psychosis): If symptoms occur in response to events that, singly or together, would be markedly stressful to almost anyone in similar circumstances in the individual's culture.

Without marked stressor(s): If symptoms do not occur in response to events that, singly or together, would be markedly stressful to almost anyone in similar circumstances in the individual's culture.

With postpartum onset: If onset is during pregnancy or within 4 weeks postpartum.

Specify if:

With catatonia (refer to the criteria for catatonia associated with another mental disorder, [DSM-5] pp. 119–120, for definition)

Specify current severity:

Severity is rated by a quantitative assessment of the primary symptoms of psychosis, including delusions, hallucinations, disorganized speech, abnormal psychomotor behavior, and negative symptoms. Each of these symptoms may be rated for its current severity (most severe in the last 7 days) on a 5-point scale ranging from 0 (not present) to 4 (present and severe). (See Clinician-Rated Dimensions of Psychosis Symptom Severity in the [DSM-5] chapter "Assessment Measures.")

Note: Diagnosis of brief psychotic disorder can be made without using this severity specifier.

Box 6–2.   DSM-5 Diagnostic Criteria for Schizophreniform Disorder

---

A. Two (or more) of the following, each present for a significant portion of time during a 1-month period (or less if successfully treated). At least one of these must be (1), (2), or (3):

1. Delusions.
2. Hallucinations.
3. Disorganized speech (e.g., frequent derailment or incoherence).
4. Grossly disorganized or catatonic behavior.
5. Negative symptoms (i.e., diminished emotional expression or avolition).

B. An episode of the disorder lasts at least 1 month but less than 6 months. When the diagnosis must be made without waiting for recovery, it should be qualified as "provisional."

C. Schizoaffective disorder and depressive or bipolar disorder with psychotic features have been ruled out because either 1) no major depressive or manic episodes have occurred concurrently with the active-phase symptoms, or 2) if mood episodes have occurred during active-phase symptoms, they have been present for a minority of the total duration of the active and residual periods of the illness.

D. The disturbance is not attributable to the physiological effects of a substance (e.g., a drug of abuse, a medication) or another medical condition.

Specify if:

With good prognostic features: This specifier requires the presence of at least two of the following features: onset of prominent psychotic symptoms within 4 weeks of the first noticeable change in usual behavior or functioning; confusion or perplexity; good premorbid social and occupational functioning; and absence of blunted or flat affect.

Without good prognostic features: This specifier is applied if two or more of the above features have not been present.

Specify if:

With catatonia (refer to the criteria for catatonia associated with another mental disorder, [DSM-5] pp. 119–120, for definition).

Specify current severity:

Severity is rated by a quantitative assessment of the primary symptoms of psychosis, including delusions, hallucinations, disorganized speech, abnormal psychomotor behavior, and negative symptoms. Each of these symptoms may be rated for its current severity (most severe in the last 7 days) on a 5-point scale ranging from 0 (not present) to 4 (present and severe). (See Clinician-Rated Dimensions of Psychosis Symptom Severity in the [DSM-5] chapter "Assessment Measures.")

Note: Diagnosis of schizophreniform disorder can be made without using this severity specifier.

Box 6–3.   DSM-5 Diagnostic Criteria for Schizophrenia

A. Two (or more) of the following, each present for a significant portion of time during a 1-month period (or less if successfully treated). At least one of these must be (1), (2), or (3):

1. Delusions.
2. Hallucinations.
3. Disorganized speech (e.g., frequent derailment or incoherence).
4. Grossly disorganized or catatonic behavior.
5. Negative symptoms (i.e., diminished emotional expression or avolition).

B. For a significant portion of the time since the onset of the disturbance, level of functioning in one or more major areas, such as work, interpersonal relations, or self-care, is markedly below the level achieved prior to the onset (or when the onset is in childhood or adolescence, there is failure to achieve expected level of interpersonal, academic, or occupational functioning).

C. Continuous signs of the disturbance persist for at least 6 months. This 6-month period must include at least 1 month of symptoms (or less if successfully treated) that meet Criterion A (i.e., active-phase symptoms) and may include periods of prodromal or residual symptoms. During these prodromal or residual periods, the signs of the disturbance may be manifested by only negative symptoms or by two or more symptoms listed in Criterion A present in an attenuated form (e.g., odd beliefs, unusual perceptual experiences).

D. Schizoaffective disorder and depressive or bipolar disorder with psychotic features have been ruled out because either 1) no major depressive or manic episodes have occurred concurrently with the active-phase symptoms, or 2) if mood episodes have occurred during active-phase symptoms, they have been present for a minority of the total duration of the active and residual periods of the illness.

E. The disturbance is not attributable to the physiological effects of a substance (e.g., a drug of abuse, a medication) or another medical condition.

F. If there is a history of autism spectrum disorder or a communication disorder of childhood onset, the additional diagnosis of schizophrenia is made only if prominent delusions or hallucinations, in addition to the other required symptoms of schizophrenia, are also present for at least 1 month (or less if successfully treated).

Specify if:

The following course specifiers are only to be used after a 1-year duration of the disorder and if they are not in contradiction to the diagnostic course criteria.

First episode, currently in acute episode: First manifestation of the disorder meeting the defining diagnostic symptom and time criteria. An *acute episode* is a time period in which the symptom criteria are fulfilled.

First episode, currently in partial remission: *Partial remission* is a period of time during which an improvement after a previous episode is maintained and in which the defining criteria of the disorder are only partially fulfilled.

First episode, currently in full remission: *Full remission* is a period of time after a previous episode during which no disorder-specific symptoms are present.

Multiple episodes, currently in acute episode: Multiple episodes may be determined after a minimum of two episodes (i.e., after a first episode, a remission and a minimum of one relapse).

Multiple episodes, currently in partial remission

Multiple episodes, currently in full remission

Continuous: Symptoms fulfilling the diagnostic symptom criteria of the disorder are remaining for the majority of the illness course, with subthreshold symptom periods being very brief relative to the overall course.

Unspecified

Specify if:

With catatonia (refer to the criteria for catatonia associated with another mental disorder, [DSM-5] pp. 119–120, for definition).

Specify current severity:

> Severity is rated by a quantitative assessment of the primary symptoms of psychosis, including delusions, hallucinations, disorganized speech, abnormal psychomotor behavior, and negative symptoms. Each of these symptoms may be rated for its current severity (most severe in the last 7 days) on a 5-point scale ranging from 0 (not present) to 4 (present and severe). (See Clinician-Rated Dimensions of Psychosis Symptom Severity in the [DSM-5] chapter "Assessment Measures.")
> **Note:** Diagnosis of schizophrenia can be made without using this severity specifier.

Box 6–4.   DSM-5 Diagnostic Criteria for Substance/Medication-Induced Psychotic Disorder

A. Presence of one or both of the following symptoms:

   1. Delusions.
   2. Hallucinations.

B. There is evidence from the history, physical examination, or laboratory findings of both (1) and (2):

   1. The symptoms in Criterion A developed during or soon after substance intoxication or withdrawal or after exposure to a medication.
   2. The involved substance/medication is capable of producing the symptoms in Criterion A.

C. The disturbance is not better explained by a psychotic disorder that is not substance/medication-induced. Such evidence of an independent psychotic disorder could include the following:

   > The symptoms preceded the onset of the substance/medication use; the symptoms persist for a substantial period of time (e.g., about 1 month) after the cessation of acute withdrawal or severe intoxication; or there is other evidence of an independent non-substance/medication-induced psychotic disorder (e.g., a history of recurrent non-substance/medication-related episodes).

D. The disturbance does not occur exclusively during the course of a delirium.
E. The disturbance causes clinically significant distress or impairment in social, occupational, or other important areas of functioning.

Note: This diagnosis should be made instead of a diagnosis of substance intoxication or substance withdrawal only when the symptoms in Criterion A predominate in the clinical picture and when they are sufficiently severe to warrant clinical attention.

Specify if (see Table 1 in the [DSM-5] chapter "Substance-Related and Addictive Disorders" for diagnoses associated with substance class):

> **With onset during intoxication:** If the criteria are met for intoxication with the substance and the symptoms develop during intoxication.

With onset during withdrawal: If the criteria are met for withdrawal from the substance and the symptoms develop during, or shortly after, withdrawal.

Specify current severity:

Severity is rated by a quantitative assessment of the primary symptoms of psychosis, including delusions, hallucinations, abnormal psychomotor behavior, and negative symptoms. Each of these symptoms may be rated for its current severity (most severe in the last 7 days) on a 5-point scale ranging from 0 (not present) to 4 (present and severe). (See Clinician-Rated Dimensions of Psychosis Symptom Severity in the [DSM-5] chapter "Assessment Measures.")

Note: Diagnosis of substance/medication-induced psychotic disorder can be made without using this severity specifier.

Differentiating primary psychotic disorders from SIPD may be challenging or impossible during the initial evaluation of a patient with psychotic symptoms and concurrent or recent substance use. Among patients presenting with first-episode psychosis, 7%–25% are reported to have SIPD (American Psychiatric Association 2013). On evaluation of a patient with first-episode psychosis following use of or withdrawal from a substance listed in Table 6–1, an extended period of abstinence (1 month or more) with follow-up to observe whether psychotic symptoms resolve completely may be the only way to be certain of a diagnosis (see Figure 6–1). Furthermore, unless symptoms rapidly resolve during an observational period in the emergency department or an inpatient setting, antipsychotic medications should be started before the patient has completed an abstinence trial. Thus, the patient and family may not be able to discern if the resolution of symptoms can be attributed to abstinence from the substance or to the medication. For patients with long-standing psychotic symptoms, the clinician should try to determine if there has been a period of psychosis in absence of substance use (again, for 1 month of more of abstinence). A history of psychotic symptoms that are recurrent or continuous despite periods of abstinence suggests that the patient's psychosis is not directly attributable to the substance. However, DSM-5 notes that a history of a previous primary psychotic disorder does not rule out SIPD if the patient's symptoms rapidly followed substance use or withdrawal and do not fit a clear pattern from his or her previous diagnosis.

A few characteristics may suggest that an episode of psychosis is more likely SIPD or a primary psychotic disorder. DSM-5 states that psychosis is more likely substance induced in patients with an atypical age at onset (e.g., a male in mid-adulthood, an elderly patient). A recent study specifically investigated characteristics of cannabis-induced psychotic disorder and primary psychotic disorders among patients with concurrent new-onset psychosis and marijuana use (Rubio et al. 2012). The investigators found that one-third of

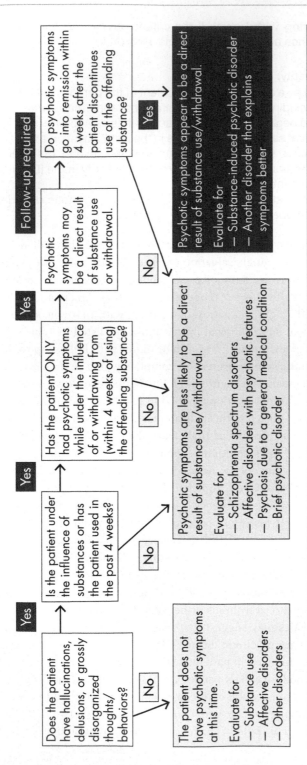

FIGURE 6–1. A brief algorithm for determining if psychotic symptoms are caused by substance use.

their sample had a diagnosis of SIPD rather than a primary psychotic disorder after a 6-month follow-up. Patients in the cannabis-induced psychotic disorder group were older, were more likely to be employed, smoked more marijuana, had greater depressive symptoms, and had more interpersonal sensitivity than patients with a primary psychotic disorder. A second, smaller study of patients with first-episode psychosis and concurrent substance use found that SIPD was associated with greater levels of marijuana use and previous trauma, whereas a primary psychotic disorder was associated with a family history of psychosis (Fraser et al. 2012).

Rates of Marijuana and Other Substance Use Disorders Among Individuals With Psychotic Disorders

It is widely acknowledged that nicotine, alcohol, and illicit drug use and misuse are more common among individuals with schizophrenia spectrum disorders than in the general population. Marijuana is the most commonly used illicit substance, and it is used more commonly than alcohol in many samples, despite legal barriers to obtaining the drug (Ramsay and Compton 2011). A review of worldwide epidemiological and clinical study samples estimated that 29.9% and 42.1% of individuals with psychosis used marijuana either in the past 12 months or in their lifetime and that 18.8% and 22.5% had either recent or lifetime cannabis use disorders, respectively (Green et al. 2005). A recent Norwegian registry–based study found similar rates of non-alcohol-related substance use disorders among individuals with schizophrenia and other mental illnesses. Individuals with schizophrenia had the highest rate of substance misuse: approximately 21%, compared with 12% and 6.5% among those with bipolar disorder and depression, respectively (Nesvåg et al. 2015). Reported rates of marijuana use among individuals who are at high risk for psychosis range from 33% to 54% (Addington et al. 2014). Although the prevalence estimates cited above may be biased by the use of clinical samples (e.g., those who are seeking medical attention), they are notably higher than reported rates of marijuana use in the general population. Recent epidemiological data suggest that 1.6%–14.8% of the population between ages 18 and 64 years have used marijuana in the past year, with highest rates of use in North America, Central and Western Africa, and Oceania (United Nations Office on Drugs and Crime 2011).

Motivations for Marijuana Use Among Individuals With Psychotic Disorders

Understanding the motivations for marijuana use among individuals with psychosis helps clinicians work with patients to decrease abuse of this and other substances and also helps them understand why this behavior is associated with psychosis. Numerous qualitative and quantitative studies have been conducted to this end and were reviewed systematically by Dekker et al. (2009). Across five studies from diverse settings, individuals with psychotic disorders most commonly reported the following motivations for marijuana use:

1. *Dysphoria relief*: Some 66.3% reported wanting to relax or to relieve depression, boredom, or anxiety.
2. *Social reasons*: Reasons including to "go along with the group," become more talkative, and have something to do with friends were reported by 61.7%.
3. *Enhancement of positive affect or enjoyment*: 42.1% reported wanting to "get high" or taking marijuana for pleasure or entertainment or to feel good about themselves.
4. *Illness- or medication-related reasons*: Only 12.9% reported a reason in this category, such as to decrease hallucinations or paranoia, or to relieve a sense of "slowed thinking" from their medications.

By comparison, a survey of more than 600 recent high school graduates in the United States who reported using marijuana found that the most frequently endorsed motivations for using marijuana included enjoyment (52.1%), conformity or social enhancement (42.8% and 25.7%), and experimentation (41.2%). Although dysphoria relief was not reported in aggregate in this study, primary reasons for marijuana use included motivations in this category, such as boredom (25.1%), relaxation (24.6%), and coping with stress or depression (18.1%) (Lee et al. 2007). There is considerable overlap in the motivations for marijuana use among individuals with schizophrenia with this sample of presumably healthy young adults, albeit with more emphasis on dysphoria relief and less on experimentation.

Marijuana Use and the Pathogenesis of Psychotic Disorders

There exists a long and complex history of understanding and acceptance of the potential connection between marijuana use and the etiology of psychosis and psychotic disorders. Historically, this potential connection has at times been exaggerated (e.g., in the era of *Reefer Madness* propaganda). Today, many advocates for the legalization of medical marijuana and recreational marijuana deny any evidence of an etiological link. Putting the history of extremes aside, here we present the current evidence of the association between marijuana use and the etiology of schizophrenia and related psychotic disorders.

Marijuana Use and Increased Risk of Developing Psychotic Disorders

There is overwhelming evidence from cohort studies in Europe, North America, and Australasia that marijuana use is associated with increased risk for later developing a psychotic disorder. Semple et al. (2005) conducted a systematic review and meta-analysis of cross-sectional and prospective studies examining the relationship between marijuana use and psychosis. They concluded that marijuana use is an independent risk factor for psychosis, with a pooled odds ratio (OR) of 2.9 (95% confidence interval [CI] = 2.4–3.6). A second systematic review of 35 longitudinal population-based studies found an increased risk of any psychotic outcome (independent of transient effects) in individuals who had ever used marijuana, with a pooled adjusted OR of 1.4 (95% CI = 1.2–1.6) (Moore et al. 2007). Both reviews noted a dose-response effect across the included studies.

Directionality of the Marijuana-Psychosis Association

Multiple theories have been proposed to explain the high rates of comorbid marijuana use and psychosis. Five hypotheses about the relationship between marijuana use and schizophrenia have been proposed (Smit et al. 2004):

1. *The self-medication hypothesis*: that people with schizophrenia use marijuana to relieve the symptoms of their illness
2. *The co-occurring drug use hypothesis*: that people who use marijuana are then more likely to use other "hard" drugs and that these other drugs contribute to the risk of developing schizophrenia
3. *The confounding hypothesis*: that a third factor increases the risk of both marijuana use and schizophrenia
4. *The interaction hypothesis*: that marijuana use increases risk of schizophrenia but only in groups with an underlying vulnerability
5. *The etiological hypothesis*: that marijuana use makes a unique contribution to the risk of developing schizophrenia

In a review of five population-based longitudinal studies, Smit et al. (2004) concluded that the evidence at that time did not support the first two hypotheses, that more research was needed to rule out potential confounding effects, and that the latter two hypotheses were both partly supported. The evidence for the first and third theories will be reviewed in the subsection "Alternative Explanations for the Link Between Marijuana and Schizophrenia," and the evidence for the latter two will be reviewed in the subsection "Marijuana Use as a Component Cause of Schizophrenia."

Theories on the Development and Emergence of Schizophrenia

The etiology of schizophrenia remains elusive but is currently conceptualized via the neurodevelopmental and diathesis-stress models. The neurodevelopmental model posits that psychosis is the end state following abnormalities that likely started during fetal growth and worsened during adolescent development (Rapoport et al. 2012). The diathesis-stress model suggests that environmental stressors can trigger pathological stress responses in individuals with biological vulnerability, ultimately resulting in a psychotic break (Corcoran et al. 2003). Research on how and why schizophrenia emerges and on how early the disease can be detected is ongoing, but the following points are fairly well accepted:

1. A number of genetic and early environmental risk factors play a role in the etiology of schizophrenia; genes and environmental risk factors may interact to affect risk.
2. Symptom onset, phenomenology, and course are highly heterogeneous.
3. Pathological changes begin before a person's first psychotic symptom occurs and continue during the early course of the illness.

Although many environmental factors, such as urban birth and upbringing, prenatal stressors, perinatal injury, and childhood trauma, have been consistently linked to a later risk of schizophrenia, not all of these factors are readily modifiable. Marijuana use, however, is potentially modifiable in the general population, in high-risk groups, and in individuals who have already developed psychosis.

Marijuana Use as a Component Cause of Schizophrenia

Given the number and size of studies on the association between marijuana use and schizophrenia, there is increasing confidence in the field that marijuana use is a component cause (i.e., one of multiple factors that contribute to the development of a disorder when combined with other causes). However, as with many factors in human behavior and epidemiological research, there is no way to conclusively test this theory. Austin Bradford Hill provided a framework for epidemiological inquiries to establish whether an association is likely causal in nature (Hill 1965), with the criteria summarized in Table 6–2. Each of the criteria will be addressed in turn.

Temporality. Data suggest that marijuana use begins before psychosis in most cases. Determining whether there is a temporal association between marijuana exposure and onset of schizophrenia is complicated by the challenges of defining when schizophrenia emerged in affected individuals. The most obvious point of reference may be the onset of frank psychotic symptoms such as delusions, hallucinations, or disorganization. However, some would argue that the onset of the prodrome is a more valid reference point for studies of causality or that genetic and environmental vulnerabilities have existed from birth. In studies that collected data on the temporal sequencing of marijuana use and psychotic disorders, marijuana use usually preceded the onset of psychotic symptoms, and in roughly two-thirds of patients, marijuana use preceded or started around the same time as prodromal symptoms (Compton and Ramsay 2009). However, there is evidence that the temporal relationship can be bidirectional. For instance, in a prospective study of a cohort of 1,580 Dutch children, marijuana use preceded (and predicted) psychotic symptoms in 32 adolescents, but having at least one psychotic symptom preceded (and predicted) later use of marijuana in 25 others (Ferdinand et al. 2005).

Consistency. The association between marijuana use and schizophrenia is remarkably consistent. This consistency in multiple prospective studies is perhaps the most compelling reason to consider this drug as a component cause of schizophrenia. In a review of seven large prospective studies, Henquet et al. (2005b) noted that this effect was observed across the board, even after controlling for potential confounders such as intelligence, baseline psychiatric symptoms, and sociodemographic variables. An association has been observed not just between marijuana use and schizophrenia but also between marijuana use and more broadly defined psychotic disorders, psychotic symptoms, schizotypy, and subclinical positive and negative symptoms in young adults (Di Forti et al. 2012).

Specificity. Marijuana use is associated with other mental illnesses, and other drugs are associated with schizophrenia, but not with the same strength or level of consistency. However, more research is needed to determine the extent to which this criterion is met.

Marijuana use is associated with depression in clinical samples from multiple studies, but the methodology of the research is sometimes lacking,

TABLE 6–2. Marijuana use as a component cause of schizophrenia: evaluating the evidence

Criterion for evaluating causality from epidemiological data	Definition	Evidence that supports the designation of marijuana use as a component cause of schizophrenia
Temporality	The factor must precede the outcome it is assumed to affect	Marijuana use begins before the onset of schizophrenia in the majority of cases
Consistency	The relationship is observed repeatedly	The association between marijuana use and psychosis has been remarkably consistent across multiple studies
Specificity	The factor influences a particular outcome or population, rather than many outcomes	Marijuana use has been associated with other mental illnesses, but not as consistently as with schizophrenia
Strength	A stronger association is more likely to have a causal component	The association between marijuana use and psychosis is small but comparable to other well-established single environmental risk factors
Biological gradient	The outcome increases with increasing exposure	In the few studies that have quantified marijuana use, increased use is associated with either a greater risk or an earlier onset of psychosis
Biological plausibility	The observed association can be plausibly explained by substantive biological explanations	Marijuana use and THC infusion cause temporary symptoms that are schizophrenia-like in nature and interact with parts of the brain that are implicated in schizophrenia

TABLE 6–2. Marijuana use as a component cause of schizophrenia: evaluating the evidence *(continued)*

Criterion for evaluating causality from epidemiological data	Definition	Evidence that supports the designation of marijuana use as a component cause of schizophrenia
Experiment	Causation is more likely if evidence is based on randomized experiments	Large-scale randomized experiments are not feasible or ethical; evaluating the likelihood of causality must be based on other criteria
Coherence	Causal conclusion should not fundamentally contradict present substantive knowledge	The designation of marijuana use as a component cause is consistent with other theories regarding the etiology of schizophrenia

Note. THC=Δ^9-tetrahydrocannabinol.

and in more robust studies the strength of the association is small (Degenhardt et al. 2012). For instance, in a household-based study of 85,088 subjects from 17 countries, marijuana use reported before age 17 was associated with depressive episodes after age 17 (de Graaf et al. 2010). Although the association persisted after local area, sex, age, tobacco use, and other mental illnesses were controlled for, it had a relatively small effect size (OR=1.5; CI=1.4–1.7) and was statistically significant in only 5 of the 17 countries. Similarly, although associations between marijuana use and bipolar disorder have certainly been reported, there is less research available on this subject. More research is needed to determine just how specific the association between marijuana and schizophrenia is. Arseneault et al. (2004a, 2004b) pointed out several studies that indicate specificity both of the outcome (schizophrenia and other psychosis-related outcomes as opposed to other domains of psychiatric disorders) and of the exposure (marijuana use as opposed to use of other drugs). Given the variability in active constituents of ingested marijuana (and their biological effects), more research is needed to determine which compound(s) has specific effects and what the necessary level of exposure is.

Strength.   Although the association between marijuana use and psychotic disorders is relatively weak, it is on a similar scale to other known single environmental risk factors. Examples of other well-established environmental risk factors for schizophrenia have similar effect sizes, including obstetric complications during birth (OR=2.0; CI=1.6–2.4) and a history of sexual abuse (adjusted OR=2.9; CI=1.3–6.4), as reviewed elsewhere (see Ramsay and Compton 2011). In a meta-analysis of prospective studies, the pooled adjusted OR of developing psychosis following marijuana exposure was 2.1 (CI=1.7–2.5; Henquet et al. 2005b). A more recent cohort study, involving 810 individuals at high genetic risk (e.g., siblings of affected individuals) and 462 healthy control subjects, estimated that marijuana users were 4.1 times more likely to develop psychosis (OR=4.1; CI=1.1–15.4). The only environmental risk factor that was stronger in this study was childhood trauma (OR=34.4; CI=4.4–267.4) (van Nierop et al. 2013). Although the added risk from marijuana use may be relatively small, the combined effect in the general population may be large, given how many young adults use this substance.

Biological gradient.   Although there are relatively few studies with adequately nuanced data to demonstrate a dose-response relationship between marijuana use and psychosis, those data that are available support this criterion. Most of the research that is currently available simply dichotomizes groups into those with or without marijuana exposure. However, when data are available, they suggest that larger doses or longer exposure to marijuana are associated with a higher risk of developing psychosis or an earlier age at onset. Henquet et al. (2005a) found a dose-response relationship between marijuana use and psychotic outcomes; in one study, the likelihood of developing psychosis progressively increased with frequency of use, ranging from 1.0 (CI=0.5–1.9) among those using marijuana once a month or less to 2.6 (CI=1.5–4.3) among daily users. Research from Spain involving individuals with psychosis (nonaffective or affective) documented a decrease in age at onset of 7, 8.5, and 12 years in individuals with prior marijuana use, abuse, and dependence, respectively, when compared with nonusers (González-Pinto et al. 2008).

Biological plausibility. The exact mechanism by which marijuana could cause or increase symptoms of schizophrenia has not been determined, but the existing evidence suggests biological plausibility. One critical piece of evidence is that Δ^9-tetrahydrocannabinol (THC) can induce transient schizophrenia-like positive symptoms (such as paranoid and grandiose delusions, conceptual disorganization, and hallucinations), negative symptoms (such as blunted affect and emotional withdrawal), and cognitive deficits (D'Souza et al. 2009). The major endocannabinoid, or normal physiological compound that binds to the same receptors (cannabinoid type 1 [CB_1] and type 2 [CB_2]) to which THC binds, is anandamide (Iversen 2012). Several abnormalities in the endocannabinoid system have been reported among individuals with schizophrenia, as reviewed in depth by Castle et al. (2012). For instance, anandamide levels are increased (as much as eightfold) in both blood and cerebrospinal fluid of individuals with schizophrenia when compared with healthy control subjects, and they may play an inhibitory, or protective, role in psychotic symptoms (Morrison 2012). In some, but not all, postmortem studies of brain anatomy, subjects with schizophrenia have greater CB_1 receptor density, including in the dorsolateral prefrontal cortex and the posterior cingulate cortex, when compared with healthy control subjects (Sundram et al. 2012). Research has yet to elucidate the mechanisms by which marijuana plays a role in the etiology of schizophrenia, but there is ample reason to consider it as a plausible mediator in the pathogenesis that ultimately results in psychotic symptoms.

Experiment. Experimental studies cannot be feasibly applied to marijuana use and schizophrenia. Although THC has been shown to induce psychotic-like symptoms in experimental conditions, no randomized large-scale trials on marijuana use during adolescence have been done, nor would these be feasible because of ethical and logistical concerns. The determination of whether marijuana is a component cause of schizophrenia will have to be made without such studies.

Coherence. Marijuana as a component cause of schizophrenia has become a well-accepted theory and is consistent with other theories regarding the etiology of schizophrenia. The role of marijuana as a component cause of this illness is consistent with the long-established neurodevelopmental and diathesis-stress theories on the development of schizophrenia. One major limitation to understanding how marijuana contributes to schizophrenia is the likely heterogeneity in the etiology leading to a constellation of symptoms that, itself, is highly heterogeneous.

Alternative Explanations for the Link Between Marijuana and Schizophrenia

Although there is substantial evidence to support the increasingly accepted theory that marijuana use is a component cause of schizophrenia, several alternative explanations for the association have been proposed and merit consideration. We will briefly review the evidence for three such alternatives: 1) the self-medication hypothesis, 2) the hastening hypothesis, and 3) the shared diathesis model.

The *self-medication hypothesis* posits that people with schizophrenia, whether experiencing psychotic symptoms or more subtle *prodromal* symptoms (those that precede the first episode of psychosis) seek out marijuana to relieve or compensate for their symptoms or to decrease unpleasant side effects of their medications. Research on the motivations for marijuana use reviewed by Dekker et al. (2009) shows that individuals with schizophrenia use marijuana for similar reasons as other adults, but there is a greater emphasis on dysphoria relief, and a small portion (12.9%) report using marijuana to relieve symptoms (e.g., hallucinations, paranoia) or side effects from their medications (e.g., slowed thinking). Ferdinand et al. (2005) demonstrated that marijuana-naïve adolescents with any psychotic symptom are more likely to begin using marijuana than those who report no psychotic symptoms. However, as reviewed by Compton and Ramsay (2009), individuals with psychotic disorders typically began using marijuana before the onset of psychosis rather than afterward. Although self-medication with marijuana to relieve the symptoms of schizophrenia spectrum disorders may occur in some cases, the available evidence suggests that this is not the primary explanation for the strong association between marijuana use and psychotic disorders.

The *hastening hypothesis* suggests that marijuana use hastens the onset of psychosis in individuals who were genetically prone to developing the disorder at some point regardless. There is ample evidence that marijuana use is associated with an earlier age at onset of psychosis. In a meta-analysis of data from 41 samples of individuals with psychosis (conducted as part of a larger meta-analysis on substance use and age at onset of psychosis), the age at onset was 2.7 years younger in marijuana users compared with non–marijuana users (Large et al. 2011). In a review of studies on psychosis conversion in individuals who were identified to be at clinical high risk, substance use was associated with conversion to psychosis in only 2 of 10 studies (Addington et al. 2014). Thus, this substance may or may not play a causative or provoking role during the prodromal period of the illness. Degenhardt et al. (2001) approached this question from an epidemiological perspective; they created mathematical models for the expected changes in incidence of schizophrenia over a four-decade period that accounted for increased marijuana use in Australia. When data abstracted from a case register in New South Wales, Australia, were compared with these models, the trends in incidence of schizophrenia during 1940–1979 did not increase at the anticipated rate based on the increase in marijuana use over the same period. The authors concluded that the data best fit either the hastening hypothesis or the shared diathesis model. However, it is quite possible that treatment, reporting, and other risk factors changed over that period, adding variability that may not be accounted for. Taken together, these data suggest that marijuana use hastens the onset of psychosis. Although some have proposed the hastening hypothesis as an alternative to the component cause hypothesis, others state that the association with an earlier age at onset merely lends more support to the latter theory.

The *shared diathesis model* purports that genetic or other factors predispose the same individuals to schizophrenia and to marijuana use or abuse. As discussed above, Degenhardt et al. (2001) argued that trends in psychotic disorders and marijuana use collected in Australia better fit the shared diathesis model than a causal model. A second piece of support for the shared diathesis model comes from the study by Ferdinand et al. (2005), described above, which found that both marijuana use and psychotic symptoms (in children with no exposure to the other) predicted the onset of the other. However, in a large prospective study, Henquet et al. (2005a) did not find that being prone to psychosis in early adolescence predicted the initiation of marijuana use, although they did find that marijuana use was a larger predictor of psychosis among adolescents with previously established vulnerability to psychosis. There is some evidence for a shared genetic diathesis for both marijuana use and psychosis, but with few exceptions, this same evidence supports the theory of marijuana as a component cause as well.

A Growing Consensus: Marijuana Use as a Component Cause of Schizophrenia

Taken together, the evidence suggests that premorbid marijuana use is a component cause of schizophrenia. Of note, it is neither a sufficient cause (i.e., it is unlikely to cause schizophrenia in the absence of other contributing factors such as genetic vulnerability) nor a necessary cause (as many individuals with schizophrenia do not have a history of premorbid marijuana exposure). The increase in risk of psychosis is small (approximately doubled) for any given individual using marijuana (Arseneault et al. 2004b). However, given that marijuana is very widely used, the impact on the number of cases of schizophrenia overall is not negligible. Some researchers now attribute 8%–15% of schizophrenia cases in some countries to marijuana use (Di Forti et al. 2012). Researchers are exploring the hypothesis that marijuana exposure interacts with other risk factors and may be particularly important in individuals with preexisting genetic vulnerabilities or other environmental insults, such as childhood abuse (Di Forti et al. 2012). At this point, it is impossible to predict which individuals are more susceptible to the effects of marijuana than others, although it is safe to say that high-risk individuals (e.g., adolescents with a family history of psychosis or who are displaying a constellation of potentially prodromal symptoms) would be well advised to abstain from using this substance.

Marijuana Use and the Clinical Course of Psychotic Disorders

Impact of Marijuana Use on the Clinical Course of Psychotic Disorders

Marijuana use after the onset of a psychotic disorder is associated, albeit inconsistently, with a variety of poor outcomes (including greater symptom severity and psychosocial problems), regardless of whether use started before or after the onset of symptoms. To our knowledge, there is only one study that administered THC intravenously in a small sample of individuals with schizophrenia and directly measured the acute effects (D'Souza et al. 2005). Although findings from this experimental data showed worsened symptoms in multiple domains, cross-sectional data on the effects of marijuana use are frequently mixed and conflicting. It is quite likely that relatively good overall functioning is necessary for individuals with schizophrenia to obtain marijuana; this prerequisite, in turn, confounds interpretation of any association between marijuana use and symptom severity or functional outcomes in such individuals.

There are experimental data from one small study and somewhat mixed cross-sectional data suggesting that marijuana increases positive symptom severity in those who already have schizophrenia. D'Souza et al. (2005) tested the short-term effects of marijuana directly using a double-blind experimental study in a small sample of individuals with schizophrenia. After administering THC intravenously, they found a transient increase in positive symptoms. In cross-sectional studies that dichotomized people with psychotic disorders by marijuana use and compared positive symptoms, several reported greater severity among marijuana users, but some failed to duplicate this finding (Bersani et al. 2002; Ramsay and Compton 2011; Tosato et al. 2013; Zammit et al. 2008). In a meta-analysis of nine studies of schizophrenia comparing marijuana users with nonusers, Rabin et al. (2011) found that marijuana users had higher positive symptom scores, even after controlling for or excluding other substance use. Regarding hallucinations and thought disorder specifically, some studies report positive associations with marijuana use, but others do not, or they find that this association is present only in those who began substance use before the onset of schizophrenia (Ramsay and Compton 2011). A number of the transient effects of marijuana in otherwise healthy individuals resemble positive symptoms of schizophrenia. The heterogeneity of cross-sectional data may simply indicate that higher-functioning (less symptomatic) individuals are better able to obtain substances.

The existing evidence is similarly mixed for negative and affective symptoms. In the aforementioned double-blind experiment on a small sample of individuals with schizophrenia, a temporary increase in negative symptoms, feelings of guilt, tension, and preoccupation occurred after intravenous administration of THC (D'Souza et al. 2005). In contrast, the aforementioned meta-analysis by Rabin et al. (2011) found no differences in negative symptoms between marijuana users and nonusers. Individuals with prominent negative symptoms at baseline may be less likely to experience the rewarding properties and may have more difficulty navigating the social interactions necessary to initiate and maintain illegal drug use. Cross-sectional data are mixed regarding associations between marijuana use and depression (Ramsay and Compton 2011). A recent large study of patients with first-episode psychosis found marijuana use to be associated with fewer depressive symptoms (Tosato et al. 2013). However, in a study of individuals with schizophrenia in France, having a comorbid cannabis use disorder was associated with suicide attempts (Dervaux et al. 2003).

Regarding the effects of marijuana use on cognitive functioning, there is, again, mixed evidence from experimental versus cross-sectional studies. Evidence from the aforementioned double-blind experiment indicated that acute cannabis intoxication results in impairments in verbal learning (D'Souza et al. 2005). However, a literature review of studies on schizophrenia and marijuana use reported that in 14 of 23 identified cross-sectional studies, marijuana users had *better* cognitive functioning than nonusers, 8 studies found minimal or no differences, and only 1 found that the non–

marijuana users had better cognitive performance (Løberg and Hugdahl 2009). Yücel et al. (2012) conducted a meta-analysis of 10 studies, including 572 patients with schizophrenia, that found better cognitive function in substance (predominately marijuana) users than in nonusers, although they noted that the included studies focused on lifetime, not current, users. They further reported data from a first-episode psychosis sample in which nonusers had greater generalized cognitive deficits (Yücel et al. 2012). Rabin et al. (2011) later duplicated this finding in 9 studies that controlled for or excluded other substance use altogether, but they concluded that the difference in cognitive functioning between the groups was not large enough to qualify as clinically significant. There are two explanations widely proposed for these seemingly paradoxical findings: 1) as for symptomatology, a better level of cognitive functioning allows individuals who want to obtain illicit substances to do so, and 2) marijuana use may cause schizophrenia to emerge in individuals who had fewer of the neurological deficits typically associated with the illness, representing a distinct etiology and possibly different clinical course.

Cross-sectional studies investigating the impact of marijuana use on health care utilization and social variables generally find that marijuana use is associated with poorer outcomes. A systematic literature review conducted by Zammit et al. (2008) found that marijuana use is consistently associated with increased risk of medication nonadherence and relapse or rehospitalization, but they note that many studies did not account for baseline symptom severity or other substance use. Substance use is associated with criminal convictions in schizophrenia and first-episode psychosis samples, as in the general population (Ramsay et al. 2011; Wallace et al. 2004).

Impact of Marijuana Cessation on the Clinical Course of Psychotic Disorders

In addition to the substantial research indicating a negative impact of marijuana use on the clinical course of psychotic disorders, studies also suggest that patients who *give up* substance use in the early stage of their illness experience benefit with regard to course and outcomes. A systematic meta-analysis that included 23 studies involving patients with psychotic disorders (Mullin et al. 2012) revealed that current substance users had higher scores on rating scales of positive symptoms and depression and lower scores on global functioning when compared with former substance users. Specifically, there was a significant improvement in ratings of positive symptoms, mood, and global functioning among patients who stopped using substances during their first episode of psychosis, whereas improvements in the symptoms of patients with a more established psychotic illness did not reach statistical significance. The authors suggested that patients in the early stages of psychotic disorders should be informed about the benefits of giving up substances earlier rather than later in the illness and that psychiatric services should consider the treatment of substance use as an integral part of the treatment of psychotic disorders.

There is also evidence that giving up marijuana use in particular is beneficial to the course and outcomes of psychotic disorders. For example, among first-episode psychosis patients in Spain, quitting marijuana use was associated with improved long-term treatment adherence (Barbeito et al. 2013). Furthermore, in a prospective longitudinal study in the United Kingdom, although changes in marijuana use were not predictive of positive symptoms, negative symptoms, or hospital admissions, reductions in marijuana use were associated specifically with reduced anxiety and improved functioning (Barrowclough et al. 2015). In a recent large longitudinal study of first-episode patients in Denmark, those who stopped using marijuana between entry and 5-year follow-up had a significantly lower level of psychotic symptoms, even after researchers controlled for baseline level of psychotic symptoms and insufficient medication dosage (Clausen et al. 2014). In a recent large study of first-episode patients in the Netherlands, persistent marijuana users had more positive and general psychopathology symptoms, worse global functioning, and more psychotic relapses compared with both nonusers and those who had discontinued their use (van der Meer et al. 2015).

Aside from detrimental effects on the clinical course per se, there are known negative consequences of marijuana use with regard to educational success, which is a crucial social domain with implications for long-term social success, physical health, and mental health, and which is already greatly impaired in many individuals with psychotic disorders. As such, marijuana-associated school problems may represent a double whammy (in addition to psychotic disorder–associated school problems) in this population. The same is true of the negative consequences of marijuana use on employment or the ability to receive and maintain benefits and entitlements; like education, employment and income sufficiency are vital for long-term success and health but are already greatly impaired in many individuals with psychotic disorders.

These findings, which pertain primarily to the crucial early stage of psychotic disorders, indicate that persistent marijuana use has adverse impacts, and discontinuation of marijuana use has positive impacts, on several key markers of both the early course and the longer-term course of psychotic disorders. As such, clinicians should consider comorbid marijuana use to be a complicating and exacerbating factor among individuals with psychotic disorders. Both psychosocial and pharmacological treatments—such as those described in Chapter 8 ("Treatment of Marijuana Addiction: Clinical Assessment and Psychosocial and Pharmacological Interventions")—should be provided alongside treatments for the psychotic disorder. Although research on treatment for marijuana misuse specifically for individuals with psychotic disorders is largely lacking or inconclusive, future research will hopefully establish the most effective treatment for this particular population.

Key Points

- Although psychosis is a core feature of schizophrenia and related disorders, it can also be caused by intoxication or withdrawal from a variety of substances, including marijuana intoxication.
- Differentiating between a marijuana-induced psychotic disorder in the context of heavy and long-standing use and a primary psychotic (i.e., schizophrenia spectrum) disorder can be difficult. DSM-5 stipulates that psychosis can be attributed to substance use as much as a month after use. To be certain that psychotic symptoms are not caused by marijuana, the patient should abstain from its use for an extended period of time to allow for determination of whether or not the symptoms resolve.
- Marijuana use is more prevalent among persons with schizophrenia than among the general population. However, persons with schizophrenia generally use marijuana for the same reasons as others—for enjoyment or relaxation, to relieve boredom, and to bond with peers.
- There is overwhelming evidence that marijuana use in childhood or adolescence is associated with the development of schizophrenia and that although the magnitude of this association is small, it is causal in nature. Marijuana is a component cause of schizophrenia: neither necessary for the development of the illness nor sufficient to cause it by itself.
- Marijuana doubles the risk of schizophrenia in adolescents who use it, but its use may be more worrisome in high-risk adolescents. It has been suggested that 8%–15% of schizophrenia cases in some areas of the world are attributable to marijuana use.
- Experimental data suggest that the acute effects of marijuana on people with schizophrenia include transient increases in symptoms and cognitive dysfunction. Cross-sectional studies on marijuana use and symptoms in schizophrenia generally show greater positive symptoms in the marijuana use groups, but mixed results for negative and other symptoms. This is likely, at least in part, because higher-functioning individuals are better able to obtain the drug and/or because the drug causes schizophrenia to emerge in people who were otherwise less impaired than those who develop schizophrenia in absence of marijuana exposure.

- Patients with psychotic disorders who stop using marijuana and other substances during their first episode of psychosis are likely to have improvements in treatment adherence, positive symptoms, mood, and global functioning. Thus, early-course patients should be informed about the benefits of giving up substances earlier rather than later in the illness, and treatment services should consider the treatment of substance use as an integral part of the treatment of psychotic disorders.

References

Addington J, Case N, Saleem MM, et al: Substance use in clinical high risk for psychosis: a review of the literature. Early Interv Psychiatry 8(2):104–112, 2014 24224849

American Psychiatric Association: Diagnostic and Statistical Manual of Mental Disorders, 5th Edition. Arlington, VA, American Psychiatric Association, 2013

Arseneault L, Cannon M, Witton J, et al: Cannabis as a potential causal factor in schizophrenia, in Marijuana and Madness: Psychiatry and Neurobiology. Edited by Castle D, Murray R. Cambridge, UK, Cambridge University Press, 2004a, pp 101–118

Arseneault L, Cannon M, Witton J, et al: Causal association between cannabis and psychosis: examination of the evidence. Br J Psychiatry 184:110–117, 2004b 14754822

Barbeito S, Vega P, Ruiz de Azúa S, et al: Cannabis use and involuntary admission may mediate long-term adherence in first-episode psychosis patients: a prospective longitudinal study. BMC Psychiatry 13:326, 2013 24289797

Barrowclough C, Gregg L, Lobban F, et al: The impact of cannabis use on clinical outcomes in recent onset psychosis. Schizophr Bull 41(2):382–390, 2015

Bersani G, Orlandi V, Kotzalidis GD, et al: Cannabis and schizophrenia: impact on onset, course, psychopathology and outcomes. Eur Arch Psychiatry Clin Neurosci 252(2):86–92, 2002 12111342

Castle D, Murray RM, D'Souza DC (eds): Marijuana and Madness, 2nd Edition. Cambridge, UK, Cambridge University Press, 2012

Clausen L, Hjorthøj CR, Thorup A, et al: Change in cannabis use, clinical symptoms and social functioning among patients with first-episode psychosis: a 5-year follow-up study of patients in the OPUS trial. Psychol Med 44(1):117–126, 2014 23590927

Compton MT, Ramsay CE: The impact of pre-onset cannabis use on age at onset of prodromal and psychotic symptoms. Prim Psychiatry 16(4):35–43, 2009

Corcoran W, Walker E, Huot R, et al: The stress cascade and schizophrenia: etiology and onset. Schizophr Bull 29(4):671–692, 2003 14989406

Degenhardt L, Hall W, Lynskey M: Comorbidity between cannabis use and psychosis: modelling some possible relationships (NDARC Technical Report No 121). Sydney, Australia, National Drug and Alcohol Research Centre, 2001

Degenhardt L, Hall W, Lynskey M, et al: The association between cannabis use and
    depression: a review of the evidence, in Marijuana and Madness, 2nd Edition.
    Edited by Castle D, Murray RM, D'Souza DC. Cambridge, UK, Cambridge Uni-
    versity Press, 2012, pp 54–74
de Graaf R, Radovanovic M, van Laar M, et al: Early cannabis use and estimated risk of
    later onset of depression spells: epidemiologic evidence from the population-based
    World Health Organization World Mental Health Survey Initiative. Am J Epide-
    miol 172(2):149–159, 2010 20534820
Dekker N, Linszen DH, De Haan L: Reasons for cannabis use and effects of cannabis
    use as reported by patients with psychotic disorders. Psychopathology 42(6):350–
    360, 2009 19752588
Dervaux A, Laqueille X, Bourdel MC, et al: Cannabis and schizophrenia: demographic
    and clinical correlates [in French]. Encephale 29(1):11–17, 2003 12640322
Di Forti M, Henquet C, Verdoux H, et al: Which cannabis users develop psychosis?, in
    Marijuana and Madness, 2nd Edition. Edited by Castle D, Murray RM, D'Souza
    DC. Cambridge, UK, Cambridge University Press, 2012, pp 137–143
D'Souza DC, Abi-Saab WM, Madonick S, et al: Delta-9-tetrahydrocannabinol effects
    in schizophrenia: implications for cognition, psychosis, and addiction. Biol Psy-
    chiatry 57(6):594–608, 2005 15780846
D'Souza DC, Sewell RA, Ranganathan M: Cannabis and psychosis/schizophrenia: hu-
    man studies. Eur Arch Psychiatry Clin Neurosci 259(7):413–431, 2009 19609589
Ferdinand RF, Sondeijker F, van der Ende J, et al: Cannabis use predicts future psy-
    chotic symptoms, and vice versa. Addiction 100(5):612–618, 2005 15847618
Fraser S, Hides L, Philips L, et al: Differentiating first episode substance induced and
    primary psychotic disorders with concurrent substance use in young people.
    Schizophr Res 136(1–3):110–115, 2012 22321667
González-Pinto A, Vega P, Ibáñez B, et al: Impact of cannabis and other drugs on age
    at onset of psychosis. J Clin Psychiatry 69(8):1210–1216, 2008 18681755
Green B, Young R, Kavanagh D: Cannabis use and misuse prevalence among people
    with psychosis. Br J Psychiatry 187:306–313, 2005 16199787
Henquet C, Krabbendam L, Spauwen J, et al: Prospective cohort study of cannabis
    use, predisposition for psychosis, and psychotic symptoms in young people.
    BMJ 330(7481):11–16, 2005a 15574485
Henquet C, Murray R, Linszen D, van Os J: The environment and schizophrenia: the
    role of cannabis use. Schizophr Bull 31(3):608–612, 2005b 15976013
Hill AB: The environment and disease: association or caustion? J R Soc Med 58(5):295–
    300, 1965
Iversen L: How cannabis works in the brain, in Marijuana and Madness, 2nd Edition.
    Edited by Castle D, Murray RM, D'Souza DC. Cambridge, UK, Cambridge Uni-
    versity Press, 2012, pp 1–16
Large M, Sharma S, Compton MT, et al: Cannabis use and earlier onset of psychosis: a
    systematic meta-analysis. Arch Gen Psychiatry 68(6):555–561, 2011 21300939
Lee CM, Neighbors C, Woods BA: Marijuana motives: young adults' reasons for using
    marijuana. Addict Behav 32(7):1384–1394, 2007 17097817

Løberg EM, Hugdahl K: Cannabis use and cognition in schizophrenia. Front Hum Neurosci 3:53, 2009 19956405

Moore THM, Zammit S, Lingford-Hughes A, et al: Cannabis use and risk of psychotic or affective mental health outcomes: a systematic review. Lancet 370(9584):319–328, 2007 17662880

Morrison P: The endocannabinoid system in schizophrenia, in Marijuana and Madness, 2nd Edition. Edited by Castle D, Murray RM, D'Souza DC. Cambridge, UK, Cambridge University Press, 2012, pp 193–197

Mullin K, Gupta P, Compton MT, et al: Does giving up substance use work for patients with psychosis? A systematic meta-analysis. Aust NZJ Psychiatry 46(9):826–839, 2012 22368242

Nesvåg R, Knudsen GP, Bakken IJ, et al: Substance use disorders in schizophrenia, bipolar disorder, and depressive illness: a registry-based study. Soc Psychiatry Psychiatr Epidemiol 50(8):1267–1276, 2015 25680837

Rabin RA, Zakzanis KK, George TP: The effects of cannabis use on neurocognition in schizophrenia: a meta-analysis. Schizophr Res 128(1–3):111–116, 2011 21420282

Ramsay CE, Compton MT: The interface of cannabis misuse and schizophrenia-spectrum disorders, in Handbook of Schizophrenia Spectrum Disorders, Vol 3: Therapeutic Approaches, Comorbidity, and Outcomes. Edited by Ritsner MS. New York, Springer, 2011, pp 289–320

Ramsay CE, Goulding SM, Broussard B, et al: Prevalence and psychosocial correlates of prior incarcerations in an urban, predominantly African-American sample of hospitalized patients with first-episode psychosis. J Am Acad Psychiatry Law 39(1):57–64, 2011 21389167

Rapoport JL, Giedd JN, Gogtay N: Neurodevelopmental model of schizophrenia: update 2012. Mol Psychiatry 17(12):1228–1238, 2012 22488257

Rubio G, Marín-Lozano J, Ferre F, et al: Psychopathologic differences between cannabis-induced psychoses and recent-onset primary psychoses with abuse of cannabis. Compr Psychiatry 53(8):1063–1070, 2012 22682680

Semple DM, McIntosh AM, Lawrie SM: Cannabis as a risk factor for psychosis: systematic review. J Psychopharmacol 19(2):187–194, 2005 15871146

Smit F, Bolier L, Cuijpers P: Cannabis use and the risk of later schizophrenia: a review. Addiction 99(4):425–430, 2004 15049742

Sundram S, Dean B, Copolov D: Postmortem studies of the brain cannabinoid system in schizophrenia, in Marijuana and Madness, 2nd Edition. Edited by Castle D, Murray RM, D'Souza DC. Cambridge, UK, Cambridge University Press, 2012, pp 188–192

Tosato S, Lasalvia A, Bonetto C, et al: The impact of cannabis use on age of onset and clinical characteristics in first-episode psychotic patients. J Psychiatr Res 47(4):438–444, 2013 23290558

United Nations Office on Drugs and Crime: World Drug Report 2011. New York, United Nations, 2011. Available at: http://www.unodc.org/documents/data-and-analysis/WDR2011/World_Drug_Report_2011_ebook.pdf. Accessed May 1, 2015.

van der Meer FJ, Velthorst E, Genetic Risk and Outcome of Psychosis (GROUP) Investigators: Course of cannabis use and clinical outcome in patients with non-affective psychosis: a 3-year follow-up study. Psychol Med 45(9):1977–1988, 2015 25654244

van Nierop M, Janssens M, Bruggeman R, et al: Evidence that transition from health to psychotic disorder can be traced to semi-ubiquitous environmental effects operating against background genetic risk. PLoS One 8(11):e76690, 2013 24223116

Wallace C, Mullen PE, Burgess P: Criminal offending in schizophrenia over a 25-year period marked by deinstitutionalization and increasing prevalence of comorbid substance use disorders. Am J Psychiatry 161(4):716–727, 2004 15056519

Yücel M, Bora E, Lubman DI, et al: The impact of cannabis use on cognitive functioning in patients with schizophrenia: a meta-analysis of existing findings and new data in a first-episode sample. Schizophr Bull 38(2):316–330, 2012 20660494

Zammit S, Moore TH, Lingford-Hughes A, et al: Effects of cannabis use on outcomes of psychotic disorders: systematic review. Br J Psychiatry 193(5):357–363, 2008 18978312

CHAPTER 7

Synthetic Cannabinoids

Emergence, Epidemiology, Clinical Effects, and Management

Marc W. Manseau, M.D., M.P.H.

Clinical Vignette:
Jason and the "Black Mamba"

Jason Chen is a 20-year-old man in his junior year of college with no formal psychiatric or medical history but with a 2-year history of bingeing on alcohol and using marijuana on some weekends. One Saturday night at the beginning of the second semester, Jason's dormitory roommate, Scott, comes home to find Jason sitting naked and confused in the middle of the room, with a bloodied right hand, most of the room's furniture overturned, and one of the windows broken. Before Scott can ask him what has happened and whether he is all right, Jason looks at him and exclaims, "Too much evil! Get out of here!" Scott calls 911, and a few minutes later, Jason is brought to the local community hospital emergency department (ED) by ambulance and police escort. In the ED, Jason is initially agitated, combative, and internally preoccupied and requires haloperidol and lorazepam intramuscularly. He is afebrile, but his blood pressure is 172/109, and his pulse is 143 beats per minute. Laboratory work reveals a serum potassium level of 2.9 mmol/L, a serum glucose level of 161 mmol/L, and a white blood cell count of 14,100 cells/μL. All other laboratory values are within normal limits, and standard urine toxicology is negative.

Jason vomits nonbloody, bilious fluid twice before becoming sedated, at which point the lacerations on his right hand are cleaned and sutured. He is given intravenous fluids with potassium repletion, and he is placed on cardiac monitoring, which shows sinus tachycardia. After 3 hours of sleep, Jason's vital signs normalize, and he wakes up. He politely asks the ED nurse, "What happened?" He complains of a moderate headache and reports feeling exhausted and that his "head is clouded." He is calm and fully oriented with no further abnormalities on physical examination, and is discharged back to his dormitory 2 hours later.

Before leaving the hospital, Jason admits that the last thing he remembers is smoking "two joints of a natural, legal incense called K2 that my friend got off the Internet." Meanwhile, as Scott begins cleaning up the room, he finds an empty foil packet with an image of a snake on it, along with "Black Mamba" and "Not for human consumption" (Figure 7–1).

To be allowed back into the dormitory, Jason has to agree to see a psychiatrist at the university student health service. On psychiatric evaluation, Dr. Fred Lee does not find Jason's presentation to meet criteria for any psychiatric disorder other than cannabis use disorder and alcohol use disorder. He provides psychoeducation about substance misuse and begins using motivational interviewing methods. They decide to meet weekly for a while for supportive psychotherapy and monitoring, which will include random urine toxicology testing per the university's policy. The treatment is uneventful— all urine drug screens are negative for 3 months—and Dr. Lee is about to recommend discontinuing their sessions in anticipation of Jason needing more time for final examinations in about a month. However, Jason presents to the next session 15 minutes late, appearing highly anxious and somewhat guarded. When he stands up to walk from the waiting area to Dr. Lee's office, he becomes dizzy and almost falls and has to grasp Dr. Lee's arm to stabilize himself. Dr. Lee gently probes whether Jason has used any substances recently, and Jason reluctantly admits to having started smoking K2 again several weeks prior to alleviate the anxiety, irritability, and insomnia that he has been experiencing since stopping marijuana and to evade random drug testing. Dr. Lee provides additional psychoeducation and encourages Jason to stop using K2 but admits that he has only recently heard of K2 and thus has limited information about its effects and risks.

Despite Dr. Lee's advice, Jason continues to use K2 on a daily basis, and by the time final exams begin, his use has increased from 1–3 grams to 5–7 grams per day. He fails to show up for three of his five final exams and fails one of the two that he does attend. Therefore, he decides to take extra summer courses to try to avoid graduating late, and he continues seeing Dr. Lee weekly. He continues to use K2 on a daily basis for another month and starts to complain more of anxiety with occasional panic attacks, as well as increasing dysphoria and trouble concentrating on his course work. Nurturing a strong therapeutic alliance and using ongoing motivational interviewing, Dr. Lee is able to help Jason stop using K2 to maximize his chances of passing his summer courses and of graduating on time the following spring. A week later, Jason presents to Dr. Lee in a highly anxious state, complaining of an escalating constellation of symptoms, including anxiety with panic and heart palpitations, insomnia, nightmares, irritability, and nausea. Dr. Lee reluctantly prescribes clonazepam 1 mg twice daily, which alleviates most of these symptoms, allowing Jason to complete and barely pass his summer courses. After the summer exams are over, Dr. Lee recommends that Jason participate in an outpatient

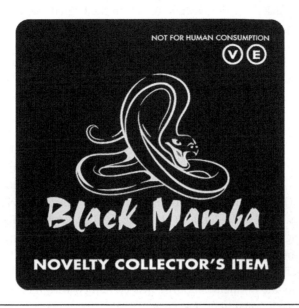

NOT FOR HUMAN CONSUMPTION

Black Mamba

NOVELTY COLLECTOR'S ITEM

FIGURE 7–1. The logo for the K2 brand "Black Mamba," from a Web site advertising its sale.

substance abuse treatment program. Jason agrees to follow through with this recommendation and expresses appreciation for the help that Dr. Lee has been able to provide.

Jason's case exemplifies several important questions about K2 and other formulations of synthetic cannabinoids (SCs), which the remainder of this chapter will explore in depth: What is K2, and where do it and substances similar to it come from? Who uses SCs and why? What is the evolving legal landscape with regard to SCs? What are the medical and psychiatric effects of such substances? How and why do the effects of SCs differ from those of marijuana? How can intoxication on K2 or related drugs and their misuse be managed? What else do we need to learn about SCs?

The Emergence of Synthetic Cannabinoids

"K2" is one of the common colloquial names in the United States for recently emerging drugs of abuse called *synthetic cannabinoids*, also sometimes referred to as synthetic cannabimimetics in the scientific literature. SCs tend to be called "spice" or "incense" in Europe and "Kronic" in Australia and New

Zealand (Zawilska and Wojcieszak 2014). In the United States, SCs are sold under numerous "brand" names, including Black Mamba, Black Diamond, Green Giant, Potpourri, Plant Food, Scooby Snacks, Dream, and Yucatan Fire, and can be purchased in convenience stores and bodegas, at gas stations, in drug paraphernalia stores called "head shops," and online (Fantegrossi et al. 2014; van Amsterdam et al. 2015). SCs are available in both powder and resin forms, but SC-containing products are most often sold as a smokable plant-based substance. The highly volatile SCs are dissolved in an organic solvent, which is sprayed on dried leaves or other vegetable matter and then allowed to dry. The plant-based material used as a substrate for smoking often contains herbs that themselves have psychoactive properties, such as wild dagga (*Leonotis leonurus*), Indian warrior (*Pedicularis densiflora*), or marshmallow leaves (Vardakou et al. 2010; Zawilska and Wojcieszak 2014). The resulting product is then sold in foil packets containing up to 3 grams of dried herbs, which are decorated with attractive pictures and written disclaimers such as "Not for human consumption" or "For aromatherapy use only." They make no mention of the SCs contained within them, but many products boast a "legal high" (Seely et al. 2012; Spaderna et al. 2013). Packets tend to be priced at $30–$40 each (Fantegrossi et al. 2014).

The first SCs were developed in the 1960s for the purposes of researching the endocannabinoid system and exploring the therapeutic potential of cannabinoid compounds (Zawilska and Wojcieszak 2014). Since then, hundreds of SCs have been identified in various samples seized by law enforcement around the world (Castaneto et al. 2014). Table 7–1 lists some of the most commonly identified SCs found in K2 and related products, grouped into five general categories on the basis of chemical structure. The first compounds were developed at Hebrew University (and thus are referred to as HU) and are referred to as the so-called classical cannabinoids because their structures are the most similar to Δ^9-tetrahydrocannabinol (THC), the main psychoactive compound in marijuana. The most commonly identified compounds include the aminoalkylindoles, phenacetylindoles, and naphthoyl pyrroles designed by J.W. Huffman, which are therefore called JWH compounds. Other SCs include the cyclohexylphenol (named CP) compounds synthesized by Pfizer, the benzoylindoles created by Alexandros Makriyannis (called AM) and by Research Chemical Suppliers (named RCS), and other miscellaneous compounds (Zawilska and Wojcieszak 2014).

The cannabinoid type 1 (CB_1) receptor is expressed extensively throughout the central nervous system (Seely et al. 2012). Most SCs have a much higher affinity for the CB_1 receptor than does THC, where they act as full, high-potency agonists, and through which most of their effects are presumed to occur. THC, on the other hand, is a partial agonist with relatively weak potency at the CB_1 receptor (Fantegrossi et al. 2014; Seely et al. 2012).

TABLE 7–1.	The most commonly identified synthetic cannabinoid compounds			
"Classical"	JWH	Cyclohexylphenols	Benzoylindoles	Other
THC[a]	JWH-007	CP-47,497[b]	AM-679	TMCP-H
HU-210	JWH-015	CP-47,497-C8[b]	AM-694	TMCP-018
	JWH-018[b]		AM-2201	TMCP-020
	JWH-019		RCS-4	TMCP-200
	JWH-051		RCS-8	TMCP-1220
	JWH-073		WIN-48,098	TMCP-2201
	JWH-081			UR-144
	JWH-122			WIN55212
	JWH-147			XLR-11
	JWH-175			
	JWH-176			
	JWH-200			
	JWH-203			
	JWH-210			
	JWH-250			
	JWH-253			
	JWH-387			
	JWH-398			

[a]Not a synthetic cannabinoid.
[b]Identified first in 2008.

SCs also have varying degrees of affinity for the cannabinoid type 2 (CB_2) receptor, which is expressed predominantly in the immune system (Brents and Prather 2014).

The first identified reports of SC-containing products becoming available over the Internet and in head shops were from Europe around 2004 (Fattore and Fratta 2011). The first SCs for distribution as spice-like products were likely resynthesized on the basis of published research reports by clandestine chemists in Central European countries, and it has been speculated that much of the current production has since moved to East Asia. The first SCs to be isolated and identified from spice products in 2008, by the European

Monitoring Center for Drugs and Drug Addiction, were the cyclohexylphenols CP-47,497 and CP-47,497-C8 (also called *cannabicyclohexanol*), and the aminoalkylindole JWH-018 (Brents and Prather 2014; Fattore and Fratta 2011). However, since these compounds were first identified, there has been a rapid expansion of the variety of SCs found in K2 and spice products. With at least 200 SCs having been identified in K2 and related products thus far, the repertoire of these compounds continues to expand (van Amsterdam et al. 2015). In addition to SCs and possibly psychoactive plant-based matter, SC products have been shown to contain numerous other compounds, some of which likely contribute to the physiological effects, including amides of fatty acids, vitamin E to mask detection of SCs, flavors (e.g., menthol, eucalyptol, vanillins), various preservatives (e.g., benzophenone, benzyl benzoate, hydroxybenzoic acid) (Zawilska and Wojcieszak 2014), sympathomimetic agents such as the potent β-adrenergic receptor agonist clenbuterol, the μ opioid receptor agonists *o*-desmethyltramadol and mitragynine, and sedative benzodiazepines such as phenazepam (Ashton 2012).

Epidemiology of Synthetic Cannabinoid Use

To date, there have been no large representative national or community-based studies of SC use, and understanding of the epidemiology of SC use is limited to analyses of case reports and case series, calls to poison control centers and ED visits, and cross-sectional surveys with convenience samples. U.S. military personnel were among the first in the country to begin using SCs, presumably to achieve a high while avoiding detection in universal random drug screening tests (Loeffler et al. 2012). In response, U.S. military branches began prohibiting SC possession and use as early as 2010 (Castaneto et al. 2014). In 2012, 10,000 random urine samples collected by the Army Substance Abuse Program that had previously tested negative for all drugs were tested for SCs, revealing a 2.5% positive rate (Castaneto et al. 2014). A Web-based survey conducted in 2011 among active duty military personnel, the Health Related Behaviors Survey of Active Duty Military Personnel, reported a 1.1% rate of SC use in the past month among 39,877 nondeployed respondents, which was higher than the rate of reported marijuana use (0.9%) (Castaneto et al. 2014). As of 2013, SCs have been included in routine military urine drug screening (Castaneto et al. 2014).

In 2013, Papanti and colleagues published a comprehensive systematic review of the clinical literature on SC use, with 41 studies meeting inclusion criteria (Papanti et al. 2013). Twenty-nine of these studies included adequate information for data extraction about individuals, which allowed for an analysis of 2,207 individuals. Confirming what had been expected from analyses of calls to poison control centers (Hoyte et al. 2012), they found that young men were most at risk for SC-related adverse events, presumably because of more frequent SC use. The analysis found that the average age of SC users was 23 years and that the male-to-female ratio for SC users was 3.16 to 1 (Papanti et al. 2013).

Calls to poison control centers about suspected SC use and SC-related ED visits have revealed a recent increase in SC-related clinical emergencies. In 2012, Forrester and Haywood published a report about calls to Texas poison control centers (Forrester and Haywood 2012). They found that during 2010–2011, 1,037 reports of SC exposure were made to Texas poison centers, from 124 of Texas's 254 counties. Population-based SC exposure rates were higher in rural counties (4.90 exposures per 100,000 population) than in urban counties (4.02 per 100,000 population). A report by the American Association of Poison Control Centers from May 2015 summarized the number of calls to poison control centers since 2011 (American Association of Poison Control Centers 2015a). There were 6,968 calls to centers in 2011, and the number of calls decreased to 2,668 in 2013 before beginning to rise again to 3,682 in 2014. As of November 30, there were 7,369 calls in 2015, which clearly puts this year on track to have the most SC-related poison control calls on record (American Association of Poison Control Centers 2015b). These data are consistent with recent reports from the Centers for Disease Control and Prevention (CDC). One report showed a 330% increase in monthly SC-related calls reported to the National Poison Data System between January and April 2015, which in total represented a 229% increase in call numbers compared with the same time frame from 2014 (Law et al. 2015). Consistent with prior data, most calls involved young men (81% men, mean age 26 years). Another CDC report, written in conjunction with the U.S. Drug Enforcement Administration (DEA), showed a large increase n confirmed SC-related adverse event reports—including deaths—between 2011 and 2015 (Trecki et al. 2015).

Results from two international online convenience sample surveys of self-reported SC users have been published. The first was conducted in early 2011 and recruited 168 English-speaking SC-using participants over 18 years old from Internet drug forums providing information about SC use (Vandrey et al. 2012). Thirteen countries and 42 U.S. states were represented. Most SC users were relatively young (the mean age at first use was 26 years), white (90%), single (67%) men (83%) with at least 12 years of education (96%). Concurrent drug use was common, especially alcohol and marijuana, and smoking was the most common route of SC administration. Curiosity was the most common reason given for use, although more than half of the respondents reported preferring the effects of SCs to other substances. About a third of the respondents admitted that they used SCs primarily to become intoxicated while avoiding a positive drug test. The second international on-line survey was conducted in late 2011 and recruited 14,966 participants, most of whom were relatively young men, 17% of whom reported having ever used SCs, and 6.5% of whom reported using SCs in the past year (Winstock and Barratt 2013). Of those reporting using SCs in the past year, 99% reported also having used marijuana, and SCs were reported to have a shorter duration of action and faster onset than marijuana. Most SC users (93%) reported preferring marijuana to SCs because marijuana created a more pleasant high and left users better able to function after use, whereas SCs caused more negative effects. However, the remaining respondents reported preferring SCs for reasons such as cost, drug-testing detection difficulties, accessibility, and psychoactive effects.

Several single-site convenience sample surveys have been conducted on SC use. In 2011, an anonymous e-mail survey was conducted at the University of Florida (Hu et al. 2011). Out of the 852 respondents, 8.1% reported having ever used SCs, a rate that was higher than for most other drugs. Reported SC use was twice as common in males and more than twice as common among students in their first 2 years. Furthermore, marijuana use was extremely common in SC users. Relationship status, race/ethnicity, and whether students lived in the dormitories were unrelated to reported SC use. In late 2011 and early 2012, 316 Australian SC users completed an online survey (Barratt et al. 2013). Most respondents also used marijuana (96%), most were male (77%), the median age was 27 years old, and 7% reported daily use. The most common reasons given for use, in descending order of frequency, were curiosity, legality, availability, positive effects, negative results on standard drug screening, and to aid in the reduction or cessation of marijuana use. In 2012, an anonymous survey of 1,740 New York City nightclub patrons was conducted to assess use of emerging drugs of abuse, and 8.2% of this sample reported SC use, which was a lower rate than had been reported in a similar sample of nightclub patrons in the United Kingdom (Castaneto et al. 2014; Kelly et al. 2013). Heterosexual identity, Hispanic ethnicity, younger age, and male sex were associated with a higher likelihood of SC use (Kelly et al. 2013).

The most representative study on SC use conducted as of the time of this writing is from the Monitoring the Future survey, which asked approximately 50,000 U.S. high school students questions that included lifetime and past-year SC use in 2010–2013 (Castaneto et al. 2014). The results showed that between 2012 and 2013, SC use decreased from 8.0% to 6.4%, whereas marijuana use increased from 23.5% to 25.8%. The decrease in SC use correlated with an increase in perceived harm from SCs, whereas the perceived harm of most other drugs, including marijuana, did not change. Further analyses using data from this study showed that female sex, black race, and religiosity were protective against SC use, whereas use of alcohol, cigarettes, illicit substances, and especially marijuana were strong risk factors for SC use (Palamar and Acosta 2015).

Legality of Synthetic Cannabinoids

When SC-containing products first became available as "natural, herbal" incense in Europe, they were unregulated. In fact, SCs were not identified in these products until 2008 (Fattore and Fratta 2011). Germany responded quickly to the identification of SCs in spice mixtures, banning CP-47,497 and JWH-018 in 2009. Other European countries, including Austria, France, Luxembourg, Poland, Lithuania, Sweden, Estonia, and the United Kingdom, followed soon thereafter with bans on these compounds (Fattore and Fratta 2011). However, subsequent analyses in Europe and Japan showed that the producers of SC-containing products rapidly circumvented such regulations by replacing the banned SCs with JWH-073 and JWH-250, thus beginning a lengthy game of legal cat-and-mouse between regulators and SC producers (Brents and Prather 2014; Lindigkeit et al. 2009).

In late 2008 and early 2009, U.S. Customs and Border Control seized a large shipment of K2 products containing HU-210, which was the first time that SCs were confirmed in the United States (Brents and Prather 2014). The National Forensic Laboratory Information System (NFLIS), under direction of the DEA, is responsible for monitoring drug use in the United States and comprises a nationwide network of local forensic laboratories, which collect and report data about drugs seized by law enforcement. The NFLIS has reported a dramatic increase in SC seizures in the United States since 2010. As a result of this data, as well as trends in ED presentations and poison control reports, 41 U.S. states have since banned sale and possession of SCs to varying extents, ranging from bans on particular SCs to bans on the entire general class of compounds (Brents and Prather 2014). In March 2010, the DEA temporarily classified the five most commonly identified SCs in the United States at the time, CP-47,497, cannabicyclohexanol, JWH-018, JWH-073, and JWH-200, as Schedule I substances (no currently accepted medical use and a high potential for abuse). However, by 2012, analyses showed that these five compounds had already been largely replaced by other SCs, such as AM-2201, JWH-122, JWH-203, JWH-210, and RCS-4. In July 2012, President Barack Obama signed into law the Synthetic Drug Abuse Prevention Act of 2012, which permanently categorized as Schedule I several known structural classes of SCs and specifically named CP-47,497, cannabicyclohexanol, JWH-018, JWH-019, JWH-073, JWH-081, JWH-122, JWH-200, JWH-203, JWH-250, JWH-398, AM-2201, RCS-4, and RCS-8 (Brents and Prather 2014).

Although SCs are now effectively banned in the United States, these regulations are difficult to enforce because of the ongoing difficulty of detecting SCs in both products and biological samples. The most common way to detect SCs is through methods employing mass spectrometry, such as gas chromatography–mass spectrometry and liquid chromatography–mass spectrometry (Brents and Prather 2014; Seely et al. 2012). Such methods are time consuming and necessitate testing for individual SCs separately. There is currently no commercially available, convenient, and inexpensive method of detecting SCs or their metabolites in serum or urine, such as the immunoassays employed in tests for other illicit substances, thus precluding the detection of all or many SCs in clinical or forensic settings (Brents and Prather 2014). In addition, although 20 countries, including the United States, banned SCs to certain degrees by 2014, the extensive Internet presence of SC producers has made it possible to manufacture SC-containing products within countries with less stringent regulation and enforcement and illicitly distribute them to a wide array of markets online (Fantegrossi et al. 2014; Fattore and Fratta 2011).

Clinical Effects of Synthetic Cannabinoids

Most of the clinical literature on the effects of SCs is made up of case reports and case series. To date, in fact, there have been no substantial, representative studies systematically characterizing the clinical effects of SC use. In addition, many case reports do not include a laboratory confirmation of SC use, and there have been very few studies describing the long-term effects of SC use (Seely et al. 2012; Zawilska and Wojcieszak 2014). However, a review of the existing literature, when combined with information from poison control reports and ED visits, suggests that SC use is associated with serious acute psychiatric and medical adverse effects and potentially deleterious longer-term sequelae.

Psychiatric Effects

Figure 7–2 depicts the psychiatric effects that have been identified after suspected or confirmed SC use. Like THC, SCs can produce euphoria and relaxation, which is presumably a main reason for its use (Spaderna et al. 2013; van Amsterdam et al. 2015). The most common psychiatric symptom that has been associated with SC use is anxiety (Spaderna et al. 2013; Zawilska and Wojcieszak 2014). Sometimes, this anxiety is similar to what has been described with marijuana use—that is, mild to moderate anxiety with milder suspiciousness or paranoia (Seely et al. 2012). However, severe anxiety with

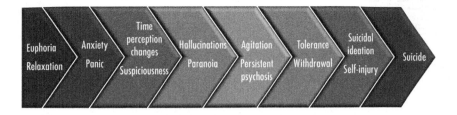

FIGURE 7–2. Psychiatric effects of synthetic cannabinoid use.

panic has also been described following SC use (Gunderson et al. 2012; Müller et al. 2010a). SC use has been associated with acute psychotic symptoms, including visual and auditory hallucinations, paranoia, altered time perception, and formal thought disorder (Gunderson et al. 2012; Papanti et al. 2013). Psychotic symptoms have been described both in people with prior psychotic disorder diagnoses and in those without such diagnoses (Van der Veer and Friday 2011; Zawilska and Wojcieszak 2014). Occasionally, SC use seems capable of causing acute agitation requiring the administration of parenteral medications and/or physical restraints (Seely et al. 2012). Acute psychiatric symptoms tend to remit with supportive care in the ED setting within several hours to a day (Spaderna et al. 2013; Zawilska and Wojcieszak 2014), but there have been cases of more extended psychotic syndromes after SC use (Berry-Cabán et al. 2013; Van der Veer and Friday 2011). Both exacerbation of existing psychosis (Celofiga et al. 2014; Müller et al. 2010b; Papanti et al. 2013) and new-onset, extended psychosis requiring antipsychotic treatment after SC use (Durand et al. 2015; Hurst et al. 2011) have been described in the literature, although the latter seems to be most often associated with repeated and/or daily SC use (Berry-Cabán et al. 2013; Hurst et al. 2011; Van der Veer and Friday 2011). There has been one case report of suicidal ideation with serious self-harm (Thomas et al. 2012) and two case reports of completed suicide immediately following SC use (Patton et al. 2013; van Amsterdam et al. 2015). Both suicides seem to have been related to severe psychotic symptoms following SC use, and in one case, the young man was found dead with multiple self-inflicted stab wounds. Postmortem blood testing identified metabolites of AM-2201 (Patton et al. 2013). There is another case report of a young man with no psychiatric history self-inflicting fourth-degree burns to both of his upper extremities after using an SC-containing product called "Black Diamond." He required bilateral amputations (Meijer et al. 2014).

Regular SC use for an extended period of time has been associated with signs and symptoms of physiological dependence, including rapid tolerance and a significant withdrawal syndrome (van Amsterdam et al. 2015; Zim-

TABLE 7–2.   Medical effects of synthetic cannabinoid use

General	Xerostomia, xerophthalmia, increased appetite, extreme fatigue, subjective cognitive slowness, headache
Neurological	Dizziness, lack of coordination, memory impairment, altered mental status, seizures, acute ischemic stroke
Cardiovascular	Tachycardia, hypertension, hypertensive urgency, orthostatic hypotension, arrhythmia, myocardial infarction
Respiratory	Respiratory depression, pneumonitis
Gastrointestinal	Nausea, vomiting
Renal	Renal failure
Laboratory	Hypokalemia, hyperglycemia, acidosis, leukocytosis, rhabdomyolysis
Mortality	Overdose death, death due to myocardial infarction or stroke, suicide

mermann et al. 2009). The described withdrawal syndrome is similar to, although more pronounced than, that of marijuana and includes craving, anxiety, irritability, insomnia, nightmares and vivid dreams, tremor, and nausea with vomiting (Nacca et al. 2013; Zimmermann et al. 2009). SCs have been shown to abort withdrawal from THC, but THC does not seem to be an effective antidote to SC withdrawal (Nacca et al. 2013).

Medical Effects

Table 7–2 summarizes the identified medical effects that have been associated with suspected or confirmed SC use. People have described xerostomia, xerophthalmia (Auwärter et al. 2009; Spaderna et al. 2013), and increased appetite during SC intoxication (Spaderna et al. 2013), and have also described "hangover" symptoms lasting up to a day after the cessation of SC use, including extreme fatigue, subjective cognitive slowness, and headache (Winstock and Barratt 2013). SC use has been associated with serious acute neurological effects, including dizziness, lack of coordination, memory impairment, somnolence or lethargy, and altered mental status (Seely et al. 2012; Zawilska and Wojcieszak 2014), and seizures in people without previously identified seizure disorders (Hoyte et al. 2012; Lapoint et al. 2011; Schneir and Baumbacher 2012). One case series described two previously healthy women in their 20s who developed acute ischemic stroke after a first exposure to SCs (Bernson-Leung et al. 2014). Cardiovascular effects have included tachycardia (Hoyte et al. 2012; Seely et al. 2012), elevated blood pressure while lying down, hypertensive urgency, and orthostatic hypotension (Seely et al. 2012; Zawilska and Wojcieszak 2014). A series of myocardial infarction cases within days of SC use have been reported in otherwise healthy young men without known prior cardiovascular disease (Mir et al. 2011). Severe respiratory depression requiring intubation has been described following SC use (Jinwala and Gupta 2012), as has pneumonitis (Alhadi et al. 2013). Severe nausea with vomiting has been repeatedly associated with SC use (Seely et al. 2012; Zawilska and Wojcieszak 2014). There have been at least several reported cases of acute renal failure after SC use, although these cases were all related to a specific fluorinated SC, XLR-11 (Centers for Disease Control and Prevention 2013; Thornton et al. 2013). Laboratory abnormalities identified after SC use include hypokalemia, hyperglycemia, acidosis, and an elevated white blood cell count (Seely et al. 2012; Spaderna et al. 2013; Zawilska and Wojcieszak 2014). There has been at least one case of rhabdomyolysis (Durand et al. 2015). There is one case report of an SC overdose causing death, although it is unclear whether the SC itself or other contaminants caused the death (Kronstrand et al. 2013). In addition, a CDC analysis of SC-related calls reported to the National Poison Data System in early 2015 reported 15 deaths out of 2,961 calls for which a medical outcome was reported (0.5% mortality rate) (Law et al. 2015). Another CDC report in conjunction with the DEA reported an increase in deaths between 2011 and 2015 associated with laboratory-confirmed SC use (Trecki et al. 2015).

Synthetic Cannabinoids Versus Marijuana

Although many of the described psychiatric and physical effects of SC use are similar to the known effects of marijuana, reactions to SCs tend to be more severe and pronounced (Fantegrossi et al. 2014). For instance, marijuana use often leads to tachycardia but usually not hypertensive urgency, and marijuana can cause psychotic symptoms but has not been frequently associated with acute psychosis with agitation requiring emergency intervention (Brakoulias 2012). In addition, as already discussed, SC use has been associated with numerous severe adverse medical outcomes that have not been linked to marijuana use, such as serious somnolence, convulsions, myocardial infarction, renal failure, laboratory abnormalities, and overdose-related death. There are several potential reasons for the described differences between the effects of marijuana and SC-containing products. Table 7–3 illustrates putative reasons why SCs may have more pronounced or severe psychiatric and medical effects than marijuana.

Because SCs are dissolved in organic solvents and sprayed onto the leaves of various plants, the actual SC content can vary widely between and

TABLE 7–3.   **Comparison between marijuana and synthetic cannabinoids**

Marijuana	Synthetic cannabinoids
Has a generally uniform concentration of THC	Wide variations between batches and "hot spots" within batches
THC is the main psychoactive compound	Specific SC compounds are widely varying and frequently changing
THC is a low-potency, partial agonist with weak affinity for CB_1	SCs are high-potency, full agonists with high affinity for CB_1
THC has limited active metabolites	SCs can have highly active metabolites
Has limited psychoactive contaminants or additives	Has many potential psychoactive contaminants or additives
May contain CBD	Does not contain CBD

Note. CB_1 =cannabinoid type 1; CBD=cannabidiol; SC=synthetic cannabinoid; THC=Δ^9-tetrahydrocannabinol

within "batches" of SC-containing products. Within-batch differences in SC concentration can results in SC "hot spots," where a single packet or even "hit" of an SC-containing product can deliver a dose of SC many times greater than another seemingly identical use (van Amsterdam et al. 2015). In addition, as already described, the specific SC compounds contained in products have been continually changing to evade legal regulation, therefore making it impossible for users to know exactly which SCs are in their product of choice at any given time; furthermore, different SCs tend to vary widely in potency (Zawilska and Wojcieszak 2014). For these reasons, it can be very difficult for even experienced SC users to anticipate or control the effects of any single instance of SC use, making overdose more likely. Whereas THC is a partial agonist with relatively weak affinity for the CB_1 receptor, most SCs are full agonists with relatively strong affinities for the CB_1 receptor and high potencies (Fantegrossi et al. 2014; Zawilska and Wojcieszak 2014). Furthermore, some SCs have been found to have active metabolites, which retain strong affinities for the CB_1 receptor and high potencies (Brents and Prather 2014; Fantegrossi et al. 2014; Seely et al. 2012). Given the fact that many SC effects are similar to those of THC but more pronounced, it can be presumed that many of the differences between the effects of marijuana and SCs can be explained by stronger and/or longer duration of action of the latter at CB_1 receptors (Fantegrossi et al. 2014). Research has shown that sinsemilla, or "skunk" marijuana, with a higher THC content and little to no cannabidiol (CBD), tends to have more adverse psychiatric effects (Di Forti et al. 2015); that CBD can reverse many of the negative psychiatric effects of THC; and that CBD likely has natural antipsychotic properties (Zuardi et al. 2012). Although marijuana may have some amount of CBD, SC-containing products do not contain CBD, thus being devoid of a potentially protective component of marijuana. Finally, whereas marijuana tends to have a fairly distinctive appearance and odor, SC-containing products are artificially created, with various additives and contaminants (Ashton 2012; Zawilska and Wojcieszak 2014). As already discussed, some of these contaminants could have psychoactive or medical effects, which may lead to unintended or even surprising toxicity.

Clinical Management of Synthetic Cannabinoid–Related Toxicity, Misuse, and Dependence

There has been no research as of the time of this writing on potentially effective treatments for SC-related toxicity, misuse, or dependence. However, case reports and case series have described interventions that have been effective in individual cases (Spaderna et al. 2013). Because the acute effects of SC use seem to last less than 24 hours in most cases, monitoring and supportive treatment are most often adequate (Zawilska and Wojcieszak 2014). For acute anxiety with panic or agitation, the use of oral or parenteral benzodiazepines is most appropriate and has the added advantages of providing prophylaxis against seizures and relieving nausea, both of which often accompany SC use (Spaderna et al. 2013). For severe agitation or more extended psychotic symptoms, antipsychotic treatment may be necessary (Spaderna et al. 2013), but it is important to note that many antipsychotics can lower the seizure threshold and increase the risk of cardiac arrhythmia, so vigilant medical monitoring should be implemented if they are used. As opposed to marijuana use, suspected SC use should in many cases increase suspicion for potentially serious medical complications. Therefore, laboratory tests should be conducted when SC use is suspected, including complete blood count, electrolyte levels, and renal function. Urine toxicology should be ordered to assess for the use of other illicit substances and/or to identify contaminants in the SC product. Intravenous hydration and electrolyte repletion should be initiated as clinically appropriate (Spaderna et al. 2013; Zawilska and Wojcieszak 2014). For cardiovascular symptoms, an electrocardiogram should be done, and continuous cardiac monitoring should be considered; reports of chest pain should be taken very seriously.

Patients presenting to emergency settings with altered mental status should be monitored until their sensorium has cleared. Because SCs tend to create a more severe dependence syndrome, including more pronounced withdrawal than marijuana, aftercare referral to a specialty substance abuse treatment setting should be strongly considered.

Future Directions for Synthetic Cannabinoid Research

Although understanding of SCs and the consequences of their use has rapidly increased over the past decade, there remain major gaps in the scientific knowledge of SCs. Much progress has been made in identifying metabolites of various SCs and in developing laboratory tests for specific compounds (Seely et al. 2012). However, there is still no available test that is rapid, simple, and inexpensive enough for the point-of-care testing that would inform clinical care (Zawilska and Wojcieszak 2014). It would be extremely helpful to both clinical work and research on SCs to have a test or series of tests capable of identifying larger structural categories of SC compounds in serum or urine, such as the immunoassays used to detect other illicit substances. The epidemiology of SC use is underdeveloped. Therefore, it will be important to conduct longitudinal studies on SC use and its consequences in representative populations at both the local community level and the national level. In addition, the clinical effects of SC use have not been characterized in a way that allows for the calculation of rates of various outcomes and complications. A representative sample of SC users presenting to a high-volume health care setting should be comprehensively characterized and then followed over a period of time to begin to assess longer-term effects. Furthermore, researchers should systematically study the consequences of SC use in specific vulnerable populations, such as adolescents and young adults, people with specific mental illnesses, people in the early stages of psychotic disorders, and people who use other substances in addition to SCs. Although recent survey data suggesting a correlation between perceived dangers of SC use and decreased use among high school students are encouraging (Palamar and Acosta 2015), we need to understand much more about how to educate the public about the harms of SC use, thus reducing use and preventing potentially serious public health consequences. Finally, there is an urgent need to identify and develop effective medical and psychosocial treatments for both the acute toxicity of SC use and the long-term effects, including addiction and physiological dependence. Because CBD can reverse the psychotogenic effects of THC (Zuardi et al. 2012), research on this compound to mitigate adverse SC-related effects may hold promise. Although the fact that most SCs are more tightly bound to CB_1 receptors than CBD may limit the utility of CBD, the facts that many SCs have very short half-lives and that CBD may act primarily in other ways than through the CB_1 receptor may mitigate this complication. In addition, because most SCs are highly potent agonists at the CB_1 receptor, the role of CB_1 antagonists, such as rimonabant, could be explored (Roser and Haussleiter 2012; Spaderna et al. 2013). It is only through a robust and diverse research agenda that we can hope to curb the mounting public health threat of SC use and associated adverse outcomes.

Key Points

- "K2," "spice," "incense," and "Kronic" are colloquial names for a group of substances called synthetic cannabinoids (SCs). SCs were originally created in research laboratories to investigate the endocannabinoid system and the therapeutic potential of cannabinoid compounds, but they have recently been synthesized by clandestine laboratories for recreational use. SCs are most often added to plant matter and sold for the purpose of smoking.
- SC use has been increasing rapidly across many Western countries during the past decade. Young men who also use other substances are at especially high risk for SC use. Many seem to prefer the effects of marijuana to those of SCs but report using SCs because of a perception that they are safer or legal, because of their lower cost and easier availability, and/or to avoid detection in routine drug screening.
- Since 2008, many countries have banned the possession and sale of individual SCs. The United States passed fairly comprehensive legislation banning SCs in 2012. However, many SC distributors have been able to evade laws by switching from banned SCs to newer, still-legal SCs and by selling SC-containing products online from countries without SC prohibitions. In addition, testing serum and urine for SCs is still expensive and time-intensive and so not widely available.
- SCs have been found to have numerous potential psychiatric and medical adverse effects, some of which are serious. Psychiatric adverse effects include anxiety and panic, acute psychosis and agitation, persistent psychosis, tolerance and withdrawal, self-harm, and suicide. Medical adverse effects include tachycardia, hypertension, myocardial infarction, somnolence or lethargy, seizures, stroke, nausea and vomiting, renal failure, electrolyte abnormalities, respiratory depression, and death. The long-term effects of SC use are largely unknown.

- Similar to Δ^9-tetrahydrocannabinol (THC) in marijuana, the effects of SCs are mediated through the cannabinoid type 1 (CB_1) receptor. However, the effects of SCs tend to be more pronounced and dramatic than those of THC. There are several possible reasons for this difference in effects, including unpredictability of the content of SC-containing products, pharmacodynamic differences, pharmacokinetic differences, and lack of protective compounds, such as cannabidiol, in SCs.
- Scientists and clinicians know very little about the management of SC use, other than that supportive measures are helpful in the acute and subacute settings. We need a robust and diverse research agenda in order to curb the mounting public health threat of SC use and associated adverse outcomes.

References

Alhadi S, Tiwari A, Vohra R, et al: High times, low sats: diffuse pulmonary infiltrates associated with chronic synthetic cannabinoid use. J Med Toxicol 9(2):199–206, 2013 23539384

American Association of Poison Control Centers: Synthetic Marijuana Data, May 19, 2015. Alexandria, VA, American Association of Poison Control Centers, 2015a. Available at: https://aapcc.s3.amazonaws.com/files/library/Syn_Marijuana_Web_Data_through_5.19.15.pdf Accessed May 20, 2015.

American Association of Poison Control Centers: Synthetic Cannabinoids. Alexandria, VA, American Association of Poison Control Centers, 2015b. Available at: www.aapcc.org/alerts/synthetic-cannabinoids. Accessed December 2, 2015.

Ashton JC: Synthetic cannabinoids as drugs of abuse. Curr Drug Abuse Rev 5(2):158–168, 2012 22530798

Auwärter V, Dresen S, Weinmann W, et al: 'Spice' and other herbal blends: harmless incense or cannabinoid designer drugs? J Mass Spectrom 44(5):832–837, 2009 19189348

Barratt MJ, Cakic V, Lenton S: Patterns of synthetic cannabinoid use in Australia. Drug Alcohol Rev 32(2):141–146, 2013 23043552

Bernson-Leung ME, Leung LY, Kumar S: Synthetic cannabis and acute ischemic stroke. J Stroke Cerebrovasc Dis 23(5):1239–1241, 2014 24119618

Berry-Cabán CS, Ee J, Ingram V, et al: Synthetic cannabinoid overdose in a 20-year-old male US soldier. Subst Abus 34(1):70–72, 2013 23327506

Brakoulias V: Products containing synthetic cannabinoids and psychosis. Aust N Z J Psychiatry 46(3):281–282, 2012 22391292

Brents LK, Prather PL: The K2/Spice phenomenon: emergence, identification, legislation and metabolic characterization of synthetic cannabinoids in herbal incense products. Drug Metab Rev 46(1):72–85, 2014 24063277

Castaneto MS, Gorelick DA, Desrosiers NA, et al: Synthetic cannabinoids: epidemiology, pharmacodynamics, and clinical implications. Drug Alcohol Depend 144:12–41, 2014 25220897

Celofiga A, Koprivsek J, Klavz J: Use of synthetic cannabinoids in patients with psychotic disorders: case series. J Dual Diagn 10(3):168–173, 2014 25392292

Centers for Disease Control and Prevention: Acute kidney injury associated with synthetic cannabinoid use—multiple states, 2012. MMWR Morb Mortal Wkly Rep 62(6):93–98, 2013 23407124

Di Forti M, Marconi A, Carra E, et al: Proportion of patients in south London with first-episode psychosis attributable to use of high potency cannabis: a case-control study. Lancet Psychiatry 2(3):233–238, 2015 26359901

Durand D, Delgado LL, de la Parra-Pellot DM, et al: Psychosis and severe rhabdomyolysis associated with synthetic cannabinoid use: a case report. Clin Schizophr Relat Psychoses 8(4):205–208, 2015 23518784

Fantegrossi WE, Moran JH, Radominska-Pandya A, et al: Distinct pharmacology and metabolism of K2 synthetic cannabinoids compared to Δ(9)-THC: mechanism underlying greater toxicity? Life Sci 97(1):45–54, 2014 24084047

Fattore L, Fratta W: Beyond THC: the new generation of cannabinoid designer drugs. Front Behav Neurosci 5:60–71, 2011 22007163

Forrester MB, Haywood T: Geographic distribution of synthetic cannabinoid exposures reported to Texas poison centers. Am J Drug Alcohol Abuse 38(6):603–608, 2012 22571605

Gunderson EW, Haughey HM, Ait-Daoud N, et al: "Spice" and "K2" herbal highs: a case series and systematic review of the clinical effects and biopsychosocial implications of synthetic cannabinoid use in humans. Am J Addict 21(4):320–326, 2012 22691010

Hoyte CO, Jacob J, Monte AA, et al: A characterization of synthetic cannabinoid exposures reported to the National Poison Data System in 2010. Ann Emerg Med 60(4):435–438, 2012 22575211

Hu X, Primack BA, Barnett TE, et al: College students and use of K2: an emerging drug of abuse in young persons. Subst Abuse Treat Prev Policy 6:16, 2011 21745369

Hurst D, Loeffler G, McLay R: Psychosis associated with synthetic cannabinoid agonists: a case series. Am J Psychiatry 168(10):1119, 2011 21969050

Jinwala FN, Gupta M: Synthetic cannabis and respiratory depression. J Child Adolesc Psychopharmacol 22(6):459–462, 2012 23234589

Kelly BC, Wells BE, Pawson M, et al: Novel psychoactive drug use among younger adults involved in US nightlife scenes. Drug Alcohol Rev 32(6):588–593, 2013 23795887

Kronstrand R, Roman M, Andersson M, et al: Toxicological findings of synthetic cannabinoids in recreational users. J Anal Toxicol 37(8):534–541, 2013 23970540

Lapoint J, James LP, Moran CL, et al: Severe toxicity following synthetic cannabinoid ingestion. Clin Toxicol (Phila) 49(8):760–764, 2011 21970775

Law R, Schier J, Martin C, et al: Notes from the field: increase in reported adverse health effects related to synthetic cannabinoid use—United States, January–May 2015. MMWR Morb Mortal Wkly Rep 64(22):618–619, 2015 26068566

Lindigkeit R, Boehme A, Eiserloh I, et al: Spice: a never ending story? Forensic Sci Int 191(1–3):58–63, 2009 19589652

Loeffler G, Hurst D, Penn A, et al: Spice, bath salts, and the U.S. military: the emergence of synthetic cannabinoid receptor agonists and cathinones in the U.S. armed forces. Mil Med 177(9):1041–1048, 2012 23025133

Meijer KA, Russo RR, Adhvaryu DV: Smoking synthetic marijuana leads to self-mutilation requiring bilateral amputations. Orthopedics 37(4):e391–e394, 2014 24762846

Mir A, Obafemi A, Young A, et al: Myocardial infarction associated with use of the synthetic cannabinoid K2. Pediatrics 128(6):e1622–e1627, 2011

Müller H, Huttner HB, Köhrmann M, et al: Panic attack after spice abuse in a patient with ADHD. Pharmacopsychiatry 43(4):152–153, 2010a 20127596

Müller H, Sperling W, Köhrmann M, et al: The synthetic cannabinoid Spice as a trigger for an acute exacerbation of cannabis induced recurrent psychotic episodes. Schizophr Res 118(1–3):309–310, 2010b 20056392

Nacca N, Vatti D, Sullivan R, et al: The synthetic cannabinoid withdrawal syndrome. J Addict Med 7(4):296–298, 2013 23609214

Palamar JJ, Acosta P: Synthetic cannabinoid use in a nationally representative sample of US high school seniors. Drug Alcohol Depend 149:194–202, 2015 25736618

Papanti D, Schifano F, Botteon G, et al: "Spiceophrenia": a systematic overview of "spice"-related psychopathological issues and a case report. Hum Psychopharmacol 28(4):379–389, 2013 23881886

Patton AL, Chimalakonda KC, Moran CL, et al: K2 toxicity: fatal case of psychiatric complications following AM2201 exposure. J Forensic Sci 58(6):1676–1680, 2013 23822805

Roser P, Haussleiter IS: Antipsychotic-like effects of cannabidiol and rimonabant: systematic review of animal and human studies. Curr Pharm Des 18(32):5141–5155, 2012 22716153

Schneir AB, Baumbacher T: Convulsions associated with the use of a synthetic cannabinoid product. J Med Toxicol 8(1):62–64, 2012 22160733

Seely KA, Lapoint J, Moran JH, et al: Spice drugs are more than harmless herbal blends: a review of the pharmacology and toxicology of synthetic cannabinoids. Prog Neuropsychopharmacol Biol Psychiatry 39(2):234–243, 2012 22561602

Spaderna M, Addy PH, D'Souza DC: Spicing things up: synthetic cannabinoids. Psychopharmacology (Berl) 228(4):525–540, 2013 23836028

Thomas S, Bliss S, Malik M: Suicidal ideation and self-harm following K2 use. J Okla State Med Assoc 105(11):430–433, 2012 23304900

Thornton SL, Wood C, Friesen MW, et al: Synthetic cannabinoid use associated with acute kidney injury. Clin Toxicol (Phila) 51(3):189–190, 2013 23473465

Trecki J, Gerona RR, Schwartz MD: Synthetic cannabinoid-related illnesses and deaths. N Engl J Med 373(2):103–107, 2015 26154784 van Amsterdam J, Brunt T, van den Brink W: The adverse health effects of synthetic cannabinoids with emphasis on psychosis-like effects. J Psychopharmacol 29(3):254–263, 2015 25586398

Van der Veer N, Friday J: Persistent psychosis following the use of Spice. Schizophr Res 130(1–3):285–286, 2011 21602030

Vandrey R, Dunn KE, Fry JA, et al: A survey study to characterize use of Spice products (synthetic cannabinoids). Drug Alcohol Depend 120(1–3):238–241, 2012 21835562

Vardakou I, Pistos C, Spiliopoulou Ch: Spice drugs as a new trend: mode of action, identification and legislation. Toxicol Lett 197(3):157–162, 2010 20566335

Winstock AR, Barratt MJ: Synthetic cannabis: a comparison of patterns of use and effect profile with natural cannabis in a large global sample. Drug Alcohol Depend 131(1–2):106–111, 2013 23291209

Zawilska JB, Wojcieszak J: Spice/K2 drugs—more than innocent substitutes for marijuana. Int J Neuropsychopharmacol 17(3):509–525, 2014 24169044

Zimmermann US, Winkelmann PR, Pilhatsch M, et al: Withdrawal phenomena and dependence syndrome after the consumption of "spice gold." Dtsch Arztebl Int 106(27):464–467, 2009 19652769

Zuardi AW, Crippa JA, Hallak JE, et al: A critical review of the antipsychotic effects of cannabidiol: 30 years of a translational investigation. Curr Pharm Des 18(32):5131–5140, 2012 22716160

CHAPTER 8

Treatment of Marijuana Addiction

Clinical Assessment and Psychosocial and Pharmacological Interventions

Garrett M. Sparks, M.D., M.S.

Clinical Vignette: Maria Seeks Treatment for Being "Hooked on Pot"

Maria Rooney rushes into Dr. Janet Frank's office apologizing for being late; she missed her bus after she found out that her roommate would not be able to watch her 7-year-old son and 3-year-old daughter and had to make alternate arrangements. Maria is a 26-year-old woman referred to Dr. Frank by the University Health Services for being "hooked on pot." She is a sophomore in psychology with a 2.7 GPA and works almost full time at a local 24-hour restaurant chain. She presented to the University Health Services with her own chief complaint of insomnia.

After Maria settles down and starts explaining her problems, Dr. Frank learns that she feels very "on edge" much of the time, feels constantly stressed, and has very dysfunctional relationships with the fathers of her two children. She has a hard time focusing on her work or her schoolwork and feels like she is constantly making "stupid mistakes." She struggles to get much sleep because of her inconsistent work schedule (often working late shifts after her children are in bed) and usually has to smoke marijuana to fall asleep. She has vivid nightmares that wake her up, often about "things that happened when I was a kid" as well as about bad things happening to her children now. She says she was a "horrible kid" who at age 13 was kicked out of the house after she accused her stepfather of molesting her from age 8 until 13. She was then homeless and wound up "hooked on all kinds of pills," and she admits that she "had to do a lot of things I wasn't so proud of," eventually leading to her being incarcerated and placed in a residential treatment facility at the age of 17. She tells Dr. Frank, "I got lucky 'cause they got me before I started using needles, you know?" She says she was in rehab twice more after this but has been "clean from the pills" since she was 21.

She is somewhat confused when Dr. Frank asks her about the referral for her being "hooked on pot." "It just takes a blunt or two to get me down at night. Just to sleep. I don't sleep, I don't get nothing done. And I don't smoke like I used to."

She explains that she started smoking marijuana around age 11, usually with her older brother. After she was kicked out of her house, she began smoking daily, up to 4 grams, whenever she could get it, especially when she could not get pills. She could never sleep without it and said that when she was not allowed to smoke in the residential treatment facility it was weeks before she could sleep again. She was prescribed fluoxetine, trazodone, and prazosin at the time as well. She was consistently smoking two or three blunts daily, "maybe 2 grams total," most days since she started school but now smokes only at bedtime because "I can't be high around my kids." She has had no psychiatric follow-up since leaving the residential treatment facility.

Maria agrees that things have not been going well, but she is not sure where her marijuana smoking fits in. When Dr. Frank explores her feelings further, she agrees that there may have been times when it got in the way. Smoking has become more expensive now that she is "trying to play it straight," and she wants her kids to "grow up better" than she did. Dr. Frank asks Maria's permission to share some research findings about how marijuana may affect sleep, mood, and one's ability to concentrate. She thinks that she might not need to smoke if she could get better sleep and maybe talk about some of the "messed-up stuff" from her childhood with a therapist, but "sometimes it just feels good, you know?" Dr. Frank gives her information on a local 12-step program for marijuana use and some resources for emergency child care in the area. Maria says that she has been to groups like that before, but they are "just a bunch of boys trying to sell you pills and get with you." She thanks Dr. Frank for not "going all *Reefer Madness*" on her and says that she will see her again next week.

In the rest of this chapter, I will explore approaches to helping Maria reduce or abstain from marijuana.

Assessment of Marijuana Use

Almost any research article about marijuana will open with some variation of the line "Marijuana is the most commonly used illicit drug in the Western world." Addiction to marijuana follows patterns similar to those of other illicit drugs, although clinical outcomes for marijuana addiction from long-term studies may, on average, be less severe than those of other drugs. Nonetheless, some individuals experience a severe and dangerous clinical course leading to significant health and psychosocial problems. Marijuana users who seek treatment for their problematic marijuana use have typically used nearly every day for more than 10 years and have tried to quit more than six times (Budney et al. 2007).

The vast campaigns to encourage general misinformation about marijuana as a "safe" and "organic" drug that is "not addictive" and may even be "medicine" have somewhat relegated a thorough assessment of marijuana use to the background of many clinical assessments. Only a small minority of marijuana users show up to addiction specialty treatment specifically for their marijuana use. Instead, they present to medical providers with chief complaints that may not appear explicitly linked to their marijuana use. They present with chronic cough and other respiratory problems to their primary care providers. They present to mental health treatment (or their primary care providers) with symptoms of depression, anxiety, fatigue, insomnia, problems controlling anger, difficulty concentrating, or relationship problems. They present to the emergency department with trauma, accidents, or altered mental status. Adolescents present with worsening school performance; adults present with worsening work performance. They may present primarily to addiction specialty treatment for problems with alcohol, cocaine, heroin, or amphetamines, only mentioning marijuana use, and often nicotine use, almost as an afterthought to their current difficulties.

Complicating matters is the fact that many marijuana users simply do not experience any (noticeable) problems with use. The most oft-cited statistic suggests that about 1 in 10 adult marijuana users develops dependence, with probably a somewhat higher rate among adolescents. Half of daily users are likely to become dependent (Hall and Pacula 2003). Although many individuals with marijuana dependence experience the same sort and intensity of drug-related problems that users of other substances experience, our cultural narrative has bent toward the use of marijuana being as benign as having a cocktail at an after-work happy hour or a beer during a football game. Addiction leads substance users to be extremely skilled in their ability to dismiss evidence indicating addiction. Even if problems are related to marijuana use, the connection may be dismissed by marijuana users who struggle to believe that marijuana could be a problem for them when many of the friends with whom they use seem to not be having any problems (whether or not this is true). This is a significant barrier to treatment because early detection of problems related to marijuana use may prevent further escalation of such problems.

In addition to having co-occurring substance use disorders, people with marijuana use disorders are at very high risk for having comorbid psychiatric conditions (Diamond et al. 2006). In the study by Diamond and colleagues, of 600 adolescents with marijuana use disorders, many had co-occurring attention-deficit/hyperactivity disorder (ADHD) (77%), conduct disorder (74%), depression (38%), or an anxiety disorder (29%). In general, treatment of the co-occurring psychiatric disorders will improve the likelihood of reducing and abstaining from marijuana use, although marijuana use itself can create significant barriers to treating psychiatric disorders.

Screening Tools

Several valid and reliable screening tools are available that may help with the assessment of marijuana use and marijuana-related problems; such resources can be obtained online for free at the Web site of the Australian National Cannabis Prevention and Information Centre (www.ncpic.org.au). The Cannabis Use Problems Identification Test (CUPIT; Bashford et al. 2010) is a 16-question screening tool for marijuana use and marijuana-related problems that covers the past 12 months and is particularly useful for initial screening of marijuana use and identifying issues for treatment. The Severity of Dependence Scale (SDS; Gossop et al. 1995) is a brief, 5-question screening tool for symptoms of marijuana addiction covering the past 3 months. It may be more useful for longitudinal follow-up than for single screenings. The Cannabis Problems Questionnaire (Copeland et al. 2005) is a longer, more in-depth evaluation of various problems that can arise from marijuana use over the past 3 months. An adolescent version is also available that delves further into issues with parents, romantic partners, and school and work functioning.

Assessing Amounts and Types of Marijuana Use

Terminology pertaining to marijuana is highly regional and ever evolving, so clinicians should feel free to let the marijuana user teach them the meaning of various terms. Assessing the quantity of smoked marijuana is quite difficult given that strains of marijuana have such wide ranges of Δ^9-tetrahydrocannabinol (THC) and cannabidiol (CBD) content. Before interest in breeding potent strains became so popular, marijuana strains typically contained less than 10% THC, although the average THC level in an unpublished study of legal marijuana in Colorado was 18.7%, with some available strains containing more than 30% THC. Asking about preferred strains in the local area may be important for truly understanding the level of intake.

The means of consuming smoked marijuana also varies quite a bit from locale to locale and from user to user. The smallest amount that most users might purchase at a time is usually a "dime bag." A dime bag simply refers to $10 worth of marijuana, not an amount. The amount that a dime bag contains thus can vary quite a bit; at the time of this writing, it is about 1 gram of an "average" strain of marijuana. Many marijuana users buy marijuana in "eighths" or "quarters," 3.5 grams and 7 grams, respectively. An ounce of marijuana is about 28.3 grams (although many will insist that it is exactly 28 grams, based on the "eighths" and "quarters"). The amount of tobacco in a standard tobacco cigarette is usually about 0.7 grams, so an "eighth" would allow for the rolling of about 5 cigarette-sized joints of marijuana. Tobacco is sometimes added in with the marijuana. The amount that can be rolled into a joint or even a "blunt" (typically a larger marijuana "cigar") varies highly on the basis of the user. As a rule of thumb, an ounce will produce between 25 and 60 joints, depending on the strength of the strain and the rolling preferences of the user.

Besides cigarettes, smoked marijuana can also be consumed with a pipe (often referred to as a "bowl"). The amount of marijuana consumed at one time is typically similar to the amount that is smoked in a joint, although some pipes can hold much more. A water pipe, or "bong," can reduce some of the discomfort of smoking by cooling the smoke, possibly facilitating the rapid consumption of much more marijuana than might otherwise be smoked at once. Vaporizers, or "vapes," have also become increasingly popular, especially as e-cigarettes and vapes for tobacco have become more ubiquitous. They allow for the extraction of active ingredients of marijuana at lower than burning temperatures.

Marijuana extracts are becoming increasingly popular as well, and forms other than the traditional hashish oils have brought amateur chemists into more prominent roles in the development and distribution of marijuana products. Using these marijuana oil extracts is frequently referred to as "dabbing," and the various oils may be referred to as "dabs." Depending on the methods used to extract contents from marijuana plants, the resulting products may be referred to on the basis of what they resemble, either "shatter" (which looks like shattered glass), "wax" (which can look like a brownish wax), or any other evolving names for different physical forms of marijuana extracts. Because butane is a commonly used solvent in the process of making these products, they are often referred to as BHO, or butane honey oils. Rather than a pipe or a bong, these extracts are commonly consumed using a device called a "nail" or a "rig." The "skillet" portion of the rig may be heated with the nail, vaporizing the various extracts for inhalation.

Marijuana edibles have also increased in sophistication beyond just "pot brownies," and recent legalization efforts in some states have inspired rather creative forms of consumable marijuana, some of which are being mass produced and packaged in attractive ways, often to resemble currently available food products. Particularly concerning is the way that some of these edibles mimic food products that are traditionally marketed to children (e.g., lollipops, Pop-Tarts). Unlike smoked marijuana, edible marijuana products do not lead to immediate intoxication, making it much more difficult for users to "titrate" their high, sometimes leading to exceptionally high intakes that can increase risks. Also, because these edible products are not regulated by any governmental body, the information on the packaging may be inaccurate.

Clinicians should have some working knowledge of the basics of the ways that marijuana is consumed in order to comprehensively assess intake and increases or reductions in use. Given that terminology and consumption patterns can be extremely different regionally, as well as among different users, clinicians should also not assume that they know more than they do and should let the patients with whom they work teach them about the ways in which they consume marijuana.

Assessing Motivations, Triggers for Use, and Barriers to Quitting

Beyond forms and amounts of marijuana consumed, the clinician must aim to understand exactly what marijuana is doing for the marijuana user, including both what is being gained and what is being lost by continuing to use. Initial marijuana use has to serve some sort of initial function, often social engagement, and continued use tends to create a life of its own. Additionally, the assessment should allow the clinician to determine how ready the marijuana user might be for making changes in marijuana consumption.

Overall, the clinician wishes to assess what exactly a marijuana user likes about using marijuana. What the user enjoyed initially might not be what he or she enjoys now. On the basis of the principles of motivational interviewing (MI), allowing a marijuana user to discuss the positive aspects of marijuana use may also allow for exploration of aspects that might be less desirable to the user. By juxtaposing the positives and negatives during the assessment, the clinician may be able to open up a discussion of potential benefits that might come from decreasing use or abstaining entirely from marijuana, as well as challenges that may be anticipated or roadblocks that have come up in previous attempts to quit.

During the assessment, the clinician should also seek to understand in what context marijuana is consumed. Is marijuana used mostly with friends or other co-users or alone? Is marijuana used at certain times of the day, in certain locations, or in conjunction with any other habits? Are certain aspects of this context creating excessive risk for health or safety for the marijuana user? What seems to trigger cravings for use? Are certain moods or feelings prone to provoke cravings? Do certain people, including family or friends, or certain places seem to inspire use? Does paraphernalia lying around the house, or the odors of unwashed clothes or furniture, prompt cravings?

Withdrawal From Marijuana

In addition to managing triggers in their various forms, the clinician should assess the marijuana user's experience with and understanding of withdrawal from marijuana, which is frequently one of the greatest initial barriers that make reducing or abstaining from marijuana use so difficult.

The DSM-5 criteria for cannabis withdrawal can be found in Box 8–1 (American Psychiatric Association 2013). A characteristic withdrawal syndrome from marijuana had been disputed for many years and was first formally recognized in DSM-5 after being excluded from previous editions of the manual. The cannabis withdrawal syndrome is defined by the presence of three or more signs and symptoms within about a week of stopping heavy and prolonged marijuana use, suggested as either daily or almost daily use over a period of at least a few months.

Box 8–1.   DSM-5 Diagnostic Criteria for Cannabis Withdrawal

A. Cessation of cannabis use that has been heavy and prolonged (i.e., usually daily or almost daily use over a period of at least a few months).
B. Three (or more) of the following signs and symptoms develop within approximately 1 week after Criterion A:
   1. Irritability, anger, or aggression.
   2. Nervousness or anxiety.
   3. Sleep difficulty (e.g., insomnia, disturbing dreams).
   4. Decreased appetite or weight loss.
   5. Restlessness.
   6. Depressed mood.
   7. At least one of the following physical symptoms causing significant discomfort: abdominal pain, shakiness/tremors, sweating, fever, chills, or headache.
C. The signs or symptoms in Criterion B cause clinically significant distress or impairment in social, occupational, or other important areas of functioning.
D. The signs or symptoms are not attributable to another medical condition and are not better explained by another mental disorder, including intoxication or withdrawal from another substance.

Onset of withdrawal symptoms usually occurs about 24–72 hours following abstinence, reaching peak intensity during the course of the first week. Symptoms may persist for several weeks after this. Insomnia and other sleep disturbances commonly continue through the first month.

Among adults and adolescents in treatment for marijuana addiction, 50%–95% report symptoms of withdrawal with abstinence. Withdrawal symptoms make early abstinence much more difficult than previously recognized in the literature. Severity of withdrawal from marijuana seems also to be related to the severity of symptoms of comorbid psychiatric disorders. Marijuana withdrawal is neither fatal nor particularly medically dangerous.

Individuals experiencing marijuana withdrawal frequently relapse and use marijuana to alleviate symptoms of withdrawal, and they will sometimes initiate use of tranquilizing drugs to obtain relief from ongoing withdrawal symptoms. Marijuana withdrawal symptoms pose a tremendous barrier to abstinence from marijuana and other illicit substances.

Psychosocial Interventions and Motivational Strategies

Compared with the literature on pharmacological strategies, research on psychosocial interventions for problematic marijuana use and addiction consistently demonstrates that moderately successful strategies can be administered. These interventions tend to not be specifically designed for marijuana addiction but rather have been developed to address problematic use of a variety of substances, and at times they are applied to problematic health behaviors unrelated to drug use. Most psychosocial interventions for marijuana use teach or strengthen skills that can be used to either prevent relapse or decrease use. They may also aim to bolster internal motivational resources or provide external incentives for adherence to treatment plans to stop or decrease use of marijuana. Most studies of psychosocial interventions include elements or combinations of three distinct behavioral strategies, as described in the following subsections.

Cognitive-Behavioral Therapy and Relapse Prevention

The theory behind *cognitive-behavioral therapy* (CBT) is that learning processes are critical in the development of maladaptive behaviors such as drug use. CBT teaches strategies to identify, challenge, and correct problematic thoughts and behaviors in order to decrease use of drugs, enhance self-control, and support problem-solving strategies for the range of difficult situations that often co-occur with ongoing drug use (McHugh et al. 2010). *Relapse prevention* (RP) is an approach consistent with CBT that helps patients identify— and hopefully avoid or better manage—triggers for use.

A CBT therapist helps an individual to anticipate likely problems that may be faced during attempts to quit and during sustained recovery. In a directive manner, the therapist will help the individual explore the benefits and consequences of continuing to use drugs. Patients participating in CBT learn to monitor cravings and recognize them earlier so that skills and various coping strategies can be employed to reduce the risk of use or relapse. Working together, the therapist and the patient develop strategies for coping with cravings and avoiding situations that trigger cravings.

Whereas CBT is a broad-based approach that allows a therapist to target any number of issues that arise, RP is a CBT-based treatment strategy that refers to a wide range of strategies that may be effective for 1) preventing violations of abstinence from a substance and 2) preventing violations of abstinence from turning into full-blown relapse that would negate the positive recovery work that has been accomplished thus far. Early and throughout treatment, RP focuses heavily on avoiding high-risk situations and triggers that needlessly challenge self-control.

RP grew out of the work of Marlatt and Donovan (2005), who posited that addiction is best conceptualized as an overlearned habit rather than a disease and that the overlearned habit can be managed by empowering substance users to develop better personal efficacy in self-management and self-control. As a result, the habits associated with drug use can be set aside, and more fulfilling activities can replace them, leading to a more fulfilling life.

RP focuses on developing and supporting an internal locus of control and self-determination and developing the sort of specific skills that make executing self-control a more realistic possibility. The focus on specific skills has much in common with Linehan's *dialectical behavior therapy*. Because of its emphasis on a self-control model rather than a disease model, RP is not without its controversies, and as a result, its execution may be adapted somewhat to fit with other treatment strategies. RP may emphasize harm reduction when a person who uses substances struggles with abstinence or does not see abstinence as an appropriate goal.

Contingency Management

Contingency management (CM) involves frequently monitoring a target behavior and providing tangible rewards when the target behavior happens. Firmly rooted in behaviorism and classical economic theories of motivation, CM often comes in the form of token systems, voucher programs, and level systems. Methadone "take-homes," for example, are a common form of CM, and receiving cash for negative drug screens is also an example of CM. CM increases retention in treatment programs while at the same time promoting abstinence and other positive behaviors. CM programs tend toward one of two not entirely different forms, although the two have not been empirically compared head to head.

Voucher-based reinforcement awards vouchers with specific monetary or point values that can be exchanged for, in many cases, gift cards, restaurant gift certificates, electronics, movie tickets, or whatever else might be desirable and unrelated to drug use in a population. In most programs, the amounts of the vouchers increase with each subsequent positive outcome. For example, a first negative drug screen may earn $2, the next $5, the next $10, and so on. A positive drug screen would knock the reward for the next negative drug screen back down to $2. Such programs support development of self-esteem and self-efficacy, emphasize recovery as a choice that an individual can make, and maintain focus on building success. A meta-analysis of voucher-based reinforcement therapies for substance use disorders (not marijuana-specific) suggested that they are helpful for improving clinic attendance (effect size of 0.15) as well as medication adherence (effect size of 0.32) (Lussier et al. 2006). The effectiveness of the programs depended somewhat on the value of the vouchers but also on the immediacy by which the vouchers were awarded following positive behaviors.

Prize incentives contingency management awards chances to win variable prizes (often cash prizes) rather than vouchers. For example, a participant attending a clinic appointment or giving a clean urine drug screen might earn the chance to draw from a bowl for the opportunity to win a prize ranging from $1 to $100. As in voucher-based reinforcement, the number of opportunities to pick a prize may increase with subsequent positive behaviors (a second clean urine drug screen might earn three draws, a third consecutive clean urine drug screen might earn five, and so forth). A positive urine drug screen would reset the number of draws back to the original value. The combination of graduated chances for reinforcement and variable magnitudes of reinforcement may be more potent than voucher systems, although similarities to gambling have been a barrier to acceptance (of note, however, studies have not suggested that prize incentives increase gambling behaviors). A large trial from the Clinical Trials Network focusing on cocaine or amphetamine dependence demonstrated increased retention in treatment (8.0 vs. 6.8 weeks) and better attendance at counseling sessions (19.2 sessions vs. 15.7 sessions). The incentive group was more likely to achieve 4, 8, and 12 more weeks of continuous abstinence (odds ratio=2.5, 2.7, and 4.5, respectively) (Petry et al. 2005). A meta-analysis of prize incentives CM studies suggested robust short-term effects on abstinence (effect size of 0.46) that did not appear to persist after 6 months (Benishek et al. 2014).

Motivational Enhancement Therapy

Motivational enhancement therapy (MET) is a specific application of MI developed by William Miller, designed to help patients mobilize internal resources to effect behavior change by helping patients resolve ambivalence about engaging in treatment and ceasing drug use. MET was originally developed as an intervention to be tested in Project MATCH, an 8-year, multisite investigation of interventions for alcoholism comparing CBT, MET, and an adaptation of the 12-step model. In addition to the general emphases of MI, MET focuses on assessment feedback as well.

Compared with CBT, MI and MET do not attempt to guide the individual stepwise through a recovery program. MET protocols vary in the number of overall sessions but generally consist of an initial assessment battery followed by sessions guided by principles of MI. In the initial session, individual feedback is provided to stimulate a discussion about personal substance use, assess motivation for change, elicit change talk, and build a plan for change. Subsequent sessions continue to monitor progress, provide individualized feedback on progress, bolster motivation for change, and review how coping strategies are being implemented.

Miller and Rollnick (2013) have adjusted the definition of MI over the years, but their lay definition offered in the third edition of their seminal text defines MI as a collaborative conversation style for strengthening a person's own motivation and commitment to change, and their technical definition describes MI as a collaborative, goal-oriented style of communication with particular attention to the language of change, designed to strengthen personal motivation for and commitment to a specific goal by eliciting and exploring the person's own reasons for change within an atmosphere of acceptance and compassion.

The effectiveness of MET appears to vary across drug types, with the strongest evidence suggesting benefit for cessation of alcohol use but strong evidence also suggesting that MET combined with CBT is effective for marijuana use disorders. MET appears to promote engagement in treatment more than it directly produces changes in marijuana use specifically.

Effectiveness of Psychosocial Interventions for Marijuana Users

A meta-analysis of well-controlled studies of psychosocial interventions for treatment-seeking marijuana users found that the average marijuana user receiving some sort of behavioral intervention fared better than 66% of those in the control conditions for primary outcomes (frequency and severity of use) as well as secondary outcomes (psychosocial functioning) (Davis et al. 2015). Interventions included in the study were CBT, CM, and MET, as well as combinations of them. A summary of the clinical trials included in this meta-analysis can be found in Table 8–1. Overall, effect sizes for psychoso-

TABLE 8–1. Summary of the clinical trials included in the meta-analysis by Davis et al. (2015)

Study	N	Intervention(s)	Control	Results
Stephens et al. 1994	212	RP (10)	TAU (10)	No significant differences
Stephens et al. 2000	291	RP (14) or MET (2)	WL	Both tx groups>WL at 4 month follow-up. RP=MET.
Copeland et al. 2001	229	CBT+MET+RP (6) or CBT+MET (1)	WL	Both tx groups > WL. CBT+MET+RP reduced marijuana use.
Marijuana Treatment Project Research Group 2004	450	CBT+MET+TAU (9) or MET (2)	WL	CBT+MET+TAU > MET>WL. Tx groups reduced marijuana use.
Carroll et al. 2006	136	CBT+MET+CM (8) or CBT+MET (8)	TAU (8)	CBT+MET+CM > CBT+MET > TAU (more negative urines). CBT+MET+CM resulted in better attendance.
Kadden et al. 2007	240	CBT+MET+CM (9) or CBT+MET (9) or CM (9)	Supportive care	CM groups had highest abstinence during tx. CBT+MET+CM persisted.
Martin and Copeland 2008	40	CBT+MET (2)	WL	Tx group>WL, reduced marijuana use at 3 months.
Hoch et al. 2012	122	CBT+MET+TAU (10)	WL	Tx group>WL, much better abstinence post-tx.

Note. CBT=cognitive-behavioral therapy; CM=contingency management; MET=motivational enhancement therapy; RP=cognitive-behavioral relapse prevention; TAU=treatment as usual; tx=treatment; WL=wait list control. Number of sessions is given in parentheses.
Source. Summarized from Davis et al. 2015.

cial interventions for marijuana users were considered moderate (0.44). Interestingly, there did not seem to be any effect of the number of treatments employed across the studies.

Interventions With Families

Some literature on adolescents using marijuana included interventions designed to educate or engage their families in hopes of decreasing marijuana use. The Cannabis Youth Treatment Study was a multisite trial created by the Center for Substance Abuse Treatment at the Substance Abuse and Mental Health Services Administration to develop and evaluate five short-term outpatient psychosocial interventions for heavy marijuana use in adolescence (Dennis et al. 2004). Across two trials, 600 adolescent marijuana users were randomly assigned to receive various combinations of MET/CBT in different doses. One of the five arms of the trial included a family education and therapy component, and another added multidimensional family therapy. Other than cost, not much was added to the treatment outcomes by the addition of a family component.

In a more recent study, 153 adolescents with marijuana addiction were randomly assigned to receive either MET/CBT, MET/CBT+CM, or MET/CBT+CM+parent training (Stanger et al. 2015). Families were trained so that CM could be executed both in the clinic and at home, with the researchers hypothesizing that abstinence would be reinforced in the two contexts. By developing a comprehensive parenting training curriculum for the families of adolescent marijuana users, researchers hoped that families would be more empowered to intervene with their adolescents with regard to their heavy marijuana use, as well as with more general parenting issues. However, the study did not show any benefit of the addition of the parent training curriculum compared with those who received the MET/CBT+CM intervention.

Software-Based Technological Interventions

Various computer-based and mobile platform technologies may provide opportunities to adapt current interventions and to develop novel psychosocial interventions that reduce barriers to treatment and increase retention in treatment. Furthermore, technological interventions offer potential advantages such as more personalized treatments, more widespread dissemination of evidence-based treatments outside of a clinic setting, and perhaps even reduction in the costs of providing treatment.

In a placebo-controlled trial, 160 callers seeking treatment for marijuana dependence were randomly assigned to either a group receiving a telephone-based intervention consisting of four sessions of MI and CBT or a delayed treatment control group (Gates et al. 2012). Marijuana use was assessed at 4- and 12-week follow-up. The intervention was effective in reducing dependence symptoms and marijuana-related problems at both time points, and participants felt more confident about reducing marijuana use and reported a greater percentage of abstinent days at the end of the trial. In a subsequent trial involving the same population, 225 subjects who wanted to cease or decrease their marijuana use were randomly assigned to either a self-guided, Web-based intervention (Reduce Your Use), developed using the same principles as the MI/CBT phone intervention, or a control condition of educational materials (Rooke et al. 2013). Those receiving the Web-based intervention had reduced use of marijuana, fewer days of marijuana use, and fewer symptoms of marijuana abuse. The improved outcomes persisted at 3-month follow-up.

In a trial of 75 participants comparing a brief MET intervention with MET + CBT + CM delivered by either a therapist or a computer, both the therapist- and computer-delivered full interventions engendered longer durations of continued marijuana abstinence than the brief intervention and did not differ from one another (Budney et al. 2015). Effects persisted equally for both groups. The computer-delivered intervention cost $130 less than the therapist-delivered intervention, a savings that offset most of the cost of the CM component.

Although a search for mobile platform applications (apps) about marijuana will mostly yield information on obtaining, growing, selling, comparing, and preparing marijuana for use, researchers and interventionists are also creating applications on treatments to reduce use and treat insomnia in marijuana users (Babson et al. 2015).

Summary

The extant literature on the use of the most well-studied and effective psychosocial interventions in treating substance use disorders, specifically for treating marijuana use disorders, suggests that marijuana users who engage in evidence-based psychosocial interventions can expect moderate improvements in abstinence and reduction in problems related to marijuana use. Noticeably absent from the literature on marijuana use are 12-step programs. Participation in those programs for problematic marijuana use or addiction per se cannot necessarily be recommended or discouraged; however, given the frequency of co-occurring substance use disorders, the likelihood that many marijuana users would benefit from engagement in such a process seems fairly high.

Somewhat more discouraging, a review of clinical trials of psychosocial interventions suggests that the available standardized treatments are quite a bit better than not being in treatment at all, but the interventions generally do not appear to offer dramatically improved outcomes when compared with "treatment as usual" conditions. Treatment as usual is often not well defined, and clinicians providing the treatment as usual in clinical trials tend to be experienced and have training in more specific psychosocial interventions. The main issue may not be that available interventions are not effective but rather that the therapeutic action effecting change may be nonspecific. Structured interventions may serve as convenient vessels to deliver nonspecific therapeutic benefit by skilled clinicians. This is not a problem limited to psychosocial interventions for substance use and is not particularly limited to psychosocial interventions; pharmacotherapeutic agents for reducing marijuana use similarly struggle to separate from placebo when everyone in a trial is receiving the same psychosocial intervention. Still, marijuana users engaging in treatment seem much better off because of it, although even in the most optimistic studies of psychosocial interventions, relapse rates are high even among those who initially achieve abstinence.

These findings reinforce the notion that addiction to marijuana is a chronic, difficult-to-treat condition for which we have some effective tools. At the same time, more interventions are needed, more research is warranted, and there is reason to believe that the near future may offer more effective interventions that may be more easily disseminated with the assistance of technology.

Pharmacological Interventions

The U.S. Food and Drug Administration (FDA) has yet to approve any medication specifically for the treatment of cannabis use disorder or its withdrawal syndrome, although a few factors seem to be driving increased research interest in medication-assisted therapies to promote cessation of and abstinence from marijuana use. The understanding of the physical health and societal burdens of marijuana use has greatly increased. Clinicians have successfully integrated various pharmacotherapies into comprehensive treatment plans for alcohol and opioid use disorders. Also, the existence of a cannabis withdrawal syndrome has only recently come into more general acceptance, as evidenced by its inclusion in DSM-5. Cannabis withdrawal may be one of the most significant obstacles to cessation for chronic users.

Such recognition of the potential value for medication-assisted treatment has spurred a growing body of literature that may guide current or future treatment practices. Researchers have focused primarily on using medication to attenuate signs and symptoms of the withdrawal syndrome (including cravings) and to promote decreased use and abstinence. Studied medications have targeted cannabinoid receptors and dopaminergic pathways implicated in cravings for marijuana, as well as specific symptoms of the withdrawal syndrome (especially anxiety and insomnia) and underlying or comorbid psychiatric conditions that may be hindering cessation and abstinence.

Cannabinoids

Dronabinol.   Dronabinol, an oral medication that is a synthetic form of THC, has been approved by the FDA for the treatment of anorexia and weight loss associated with HIV/AIDS, as well as for refractory nausea and vomiting in patients undergoing chemotherapy. Agonist substitution therapy has been effective for other substance use disorders, mainly nicotine and opioid use disorders. Dronabinol could potentially reduce withdrawal symptoms and cravings and decrease the reinforcing effects of marijuana.

In a large 12-week randomized, double-blind, placebo-controlled trial, 156 marijuana-dependent adults were randomly assigned to receive either dronabinol 20 mg twice daily or placebo (Levin et al. 2011). All patients received weekly MET and RP therapies. At the end of the trial, there was no significant difference in those achieving abstinence during a 2-week maintenance phase (dronabinol 17.7% vs. placebo 15.6%). Treatment retention was somewhat better in the dronabinol-treated group (77% vs. 61%), and withdrawal symptoms were significantly lower in the dronabinol-treated group. Those in the active treatment group also attended more therapy sessions than those in the placebo group. Although dronabinol was well tolerated overall, adverse effects reported by the treatment group included drowsiness, feeling intoxicated, increased blood pressure, nightmares and sleep disturbances, and light-headedness.

Nabiximols.   Similarly to dronabinol, nabiximols, a specific extract of *Cannabis sativa* available as a buccally absorbed oromucosal spray, was developed as a treatment for neuropathic pain, spasticity, and other symptoms of multiple sclerosis. Each spray delivers 2.7 mg THC and 2.5 mg CBD. The delivery mechanism creates a much more rapid onset of action compared with dronabinol.

In a two-site double-blind, randomized clinical inpatient trial with a 28-day postdischarge follow-up, 51 marijuana-dependent adults were allowed to use up to 32 daily sprays of nabiximols (up to 86.4 mg of THC and 80 mg of CBD) or placebo for withdrawal symptoms over a 6-day period (Allsop et al. 2014). CBT was provided concomitantly. Overall severity of cannabis withdrawal was significantly reduced in the nabiximols-treated group, including effects on irritability, depressive symptoms, and cravings for marijuana. The treatment group also showed limited but positive improvements in sleep, anxiety, appetite, and restlessness. Retention in the treatment group was much better than in the control condition. Those receiving nabiximols did not report more symptoms of intoxication, and participants in either group could not accurately predict whether they were receiving the active or placebo intervention. There were no differences in adverse events between the treatment and placebo groups. On follow-up 28 days later, the treatment and placebo groups showed no differences in self-reported marijuana use or dependence.

Antidepressants

Selective serotonin reuptake inhibitors (SSRIs). In a trial comparing fluoxetine and placebo in a group of adults with major depressive disorder (MDD) and alcohol dependence, fluoxetine demonstrated efficacy in reducing both depressive symptoms and alcohol use (Cornelius et al. 1997). In a secondary analysis of that study looking at 22 subjects who also used marijuana, fluoxetine appeared to also decrease marijuana use (Cornelius et al. 1999).

Building on these initial data, a second trial was conducted with adolescents and young adults with comorbid MDD and cannabis use disorder. In a double-blind, placebo-controlled trial, 70 adolescents and young adults were randomly assigned to receive either fluoxetine or placebo for 12 weeks (Cornelius et al. 2010). All patients received both CBT and MET throughout the trial. After 12 weeks, both groups showed significant improvements with regard to depressive symptoms as well as the number of criteria for cannabis use disorder. End-of-study levels of depressive symptoms were quite low, and fluoxetine was well tolerated.

On the basis of the hypothesis that some marijuana users may be using to "self-medicate" depressive and anxiety symptoms, escitalopram was tested for 9 weeks in a randomized, double-blind, placebo-controlled study in 52 marijuana-dependent adults who did not have MDD or other affective disorders (Weinstein et al. 2014). Subjects also received weekly CBT and MET. Urine samples to measure THC and questionnaires measuring depressive and anxiety symptoms were collected. Of note, escitalopram was specifically chosen for this study because it is the first-line agent for moderately severe depressive and anxiety disorders in Israel, where the trial was conducted.

By the end of the 9-week trial, 50% of subjects (16 in the treatment group and 10 in the placebo group) had dropped out of the study. Data were analyzed using intention-to-treat analyses, and no differences were found between the escitalopram and placebo groups in abstinence from marijuana or anxiety and depression scores during the withdrawal or abstinence periods. The greater dropout rate in the treatment group may have reflected poor tolerability of escitalopram in this population.

Serotonin-norepinephrine reuptake inhibitors and norepinephrine reuptake inhibitors.   Given some data suggesting that venlafaxine may have greater efficacy than standard SSRIs because of its dual mechanism of action on both serotonin and norepinephrine receptors, 103 adults with co-occurring cannabis dependence and MDD or dysthymia were randomly assigned to receive either extended-release venlafaxine (up to 375 mg daily) or placebo in a 12-week, two-site, double-blind, placebo-controlled trial (Levin et al. 2013). All subjects received CBT directed primarily at marijuana use.

At the end of 12 weeks, both groups had clinically significant mood improvements (63% in the treatment group vs. 69% in the placebo group). Abstinence rates were low in both groups but were significantly worse in the treatment group (11.8%, compared with 36.5% in the placebo group). Decrease in libido was the only adverse effect reported to be higher in the treatment group compared with the placebo group. Interestingly, better depression scores were associated with lower THC urine levels in the placebo group, but THC urine levels in the venlafaxine group were roughly equivalent (and higher than in the placebo group) regardless of depression score. One theory posited by the authors was that venlafaxine may in fact worsen marijuana withdrawal symptoms and lead to more use while still improving mood despite ongoing marijuana use.

Atomoxetine, a norepinephrine reuptake inhibitor without appreciable effects on the serotonergic system, is approved by the FDA for the treatment of ADHD in children and adults. Atomoxetine increases dopamine and norepinephrine in cortical areas but does not seem to have much effect on dopamine in the subcortex, where there are fewer norepinephrine neuron terminals, putatively leading to a much lower abuse potential than stimulant medications. ADHD increases the risk for later substance use disorders, and the treatment of ADHD may be associated with decreased risk for substance use disorders, although the data on this are quite mixed.

In a 12-week double-blind, placebo-controlled trial, 38 adults with co-occurring ADHD and marijuana dependence were randomly assigned to receive either atomoxetine or placebo (McRae-Clark et al. 2010). All subjects received MI throughout the trial. The atomoxetine-treated group had significantly better scores on one of three measures of clinical status (the Clinical Global Impression–Improvement scale) but no differences in marijuana use. About one-quarter of the atomoxetine-treated group reported sexual dysfunction (compared with none in the placebo group), and gastrointestinal side effects were much higher in the group treated with atomoxetine.

Mixed-action antidepressants.   In some laboratory studies, nefazodone, with dual action on serotonin and norepinephrine reuptake as well as serotonin type 2A receptor (5-HT$_{2A}$) antagonism, has shown some significant decreases in anxiety and muscle pain during periods of withdrawal from marijuana, as well as some reduction in cravings among cocaine users. In a 13-week double-blind trial, 106 participants were randomly assigned to receive nefazodone, bupropion sustained release (bupropion-SR), or placebo (Carpenter et al. 2009). All subjects also were offered a weekly coping skills–based therapy program. Rates of abstinence from marijuana were equivalent across all three groups. Insomnia and sleep disturbances as well as irritability and anxiety improved similarly in all three treatment groups. Only 49% completed the 13-week trial, and the dropout rates were similar across treatment conditions, with most subjects failing to show up for appointments and not responding to outreach from study staff. The only two who were removed from the nefazodone treatment group for a clinical reason were for worsening of depression and worsening of anxiety. The most common side effect on nefazodone was diarrhea (8%).

Success in treating nicotine dependence and lessening cravings and nicotine withdrawal symptoms, as well as some preliminary laboratory data, spurred some hope that bupropion might be useful for alleviating symptoms of marijuana withdrawal and promoting abstinence. Bupropion-SR was also tested in the placebo-controlled trial against nefazodone (Carpenter et al. 2009) described above. Bupropion-SR, like nefazodone, did not improve abstinence or reduce withdrawal symptoms, although nearly half of the participants in the trial were lost to follow-up. One subject asked to be removed from the study because of flu-like symptoms after starting medication in the bupropion-SR group. The most common side effects with bupropion-SR were headaches (15%) and nausea (8%).

In a double-blind, placebo-controlled trial designed with methodology similar to studies of bupropion for nicotine withdrawal, 22 heavy, chronic marijuana smokers were randomly assigned to receive either bupropion-SR or placebo (Penetar et al. 2012). Participants were asked to maintain their usual marijuana usage until an established "Quit Day," at which time participants were to cease intake of THC products for 14 days. The dosage of bupropion-SR, similar to recommendations for nicotine cessation, was 150 mg daily for 3 days, followed by 150 mg twice daily for 4 days, leading up to the Quit Day. Participants also had three sessions of MET (one before Quit Day and the others on the 2 days following it).

Participants in the placebo group had significantly higher withdrawal discomfort scores as well as craving scores following the Quit Day than those in the bupropion-SR group. There were no differences in the groups on depression and anxiety inventories or sleep times. Only 9 of the 22 participants actually completed the 14-day period of abstinence from THC and were included in data analyses. Five of the 10 participants randomly assigned to the bupropion-SR group remained in the study, compared with 4 of the 12 participants randomly assigned to the placebo group. The study did not report information about those who dropped out of the study.

Anxiolytics and Hypnotics

Buspirone. An open-label study of buspirone, a 5-HT$_{1A}$ partial agonist, seemed to improve marijuana use outcomes, possibly by lowering anxiety (McRae et al. 2006), leading the same research group to conduct a 12-week double-blind, placebo-controlled trial in marijuana-dependent individuals (McRae-Clark et al. 2009). Ninety-three subjects were randomly assigned to receive either buspirone (up to 60 mg daily) or placebo. Both groups received MI throughout the first 4 weeks of the trial. Thirty-four participants were removed after randomization, mostly for never showing up to pick up the study medication. Another 9 subjects never provided any urine drug screen (UDS) data, so only 50 of 93 subjects were left for the analysis.

In a modified intention-to-treat analysis using those 50 subjects, the percentage of negative UDS results in the buspirone treatment group was 18 points higher (although the result barely missed statistical significance) compared with placebo. Self-report of marijuana use was no different in the treatment and placebo groups. There was no significant difference between the groups on anxiety measures, although decreases in anxiety did seem to correlate with more negative UDS results. Among 24 study completers, negative UDS results in the buspirone treatment group were 35% higher than in the placebo group. Dizziness was the only side effect more common in the treatment group compared with the placebo group.

Zolpidem. Difficulty sleeping is among the most prominent symptoms of cannabis withdrawal, with particular difficulties in sleep latency and sleep efficiency. Zolpidem, a nonbenzodiazepine γ-aminobutyric acid type A receptor (GABA$_A$) agonist, is FDA approved for the short-term treatment of insomnia. In a double-blind, within-subjects crossover study designed to look at sleep measures rather than abstinence, 20 daily marijuana users were randomly assigned to receive either extended-release zolpidem or placebo during a 3-day period of abstinence from marijuana (Vandrey et al. 2011). Following another period of ad lib marijuana use, the other treatment condition was applied to another 3-day period of abstinence from marijuana. Participants in the zolpidem treatment group had decreased nocturnal awakenings and improvements in subjective sleep quality. There were no differences between the treatment and placebo groups in overall withdrawal severity or cravings for marijuana.

Anticonvulsants and Mood Stabilizers

Divalproex sodium. In the first-ever double-blind, placebo-controlled trial investigating a pharmacotherapy for marijuana dependence (Levin et al. 2004), divalproex sodium was tested because of its use for treating irritability, mood lability, and aggression in various psychiatric conditions—symptoms that overlap with marijuana withdrawal. Twenty-five participants were randomly assigned to receive either divalproex sodium at a dosage of up to 1,000 mg twice daily or placebo for 6 weeks and then were crossed over to an additional 6 weeks of the other intervention. They also received CBT throughout the intervention period. On several measures, there appeared to be no difference between the placebo and divalproex treatment conditions, although adverse effects, especially fatigue, headaches, drowsiness, nausea, and jitteriness, were reported at high rates during the treatment condition.

Gabapentin. Gabapentin, an alkylated analogue of γ-aminobutyric acid (GABA) that blocks a specific subunit of voltage-gated calcium channels at select presynaptic sites, has been approved by the FDA for treatment of seizures and chronic neuropathic pain. It normalizes GABA activation in the amygdala, and such activation is thought to be related to the development of dependence on alcohol and possibly marijuana (as withdrawal from both alcohol and marijuana produces an anxious state related to increased extra-hypothalamic corticotropin-releasing hormone release in the central nucleus of the amygdala). In clinical studies (Ghaemi et al. 1998; Karam-Hage and Brower 2000; Mason et al. 2009), gabapentin decreased cravings and disturbances in sleep and mood, some of the most persistent symptoms of marijuana withdrawal that lead patients to resume using marijuana.

Chronic heavy marijuana use alters right prefrontal brain activity and impairs executive functions, including impulse control and processing of complex information. This may make it even more difficult for patients to engage in psychosocial interventions and may account for the high rates of dropping out among those initially seeking treatment for problematic marijuana use. Gabapentin has been shown to improve some of these same deficits (Salinsky et al. 2005); as such, gabapentin would be a rational choice to study for the treatment of marijuana dependence.

In a 12-week randomized, placebo-controlled, parallel-groups trial, 50 marijuana-dependent participants were randomly assigned to receive either gabapentin (1,200 mg total daily) or placebo (Mason et al. 2012). They also received weekly abstinence-oriented counseling throughout the study. The gabapentin treatment group had a significant decrease in marijuana use as evidenced by both self-reports and urinary marijuana metabolite monitoring. The gabapentin treatment group reported significant reductions in both the acute symptoms of withdrawal and more persistent symptoms such as mood alterations, cravings, and sleep disturbances. There were no differences in adverse events reported between the two groups.

Lithium. Preclinical studies in rats suggested that lithium carbonate could reduce symptoms of marijuana withdrawal by stimulating release of oxytocin, and two open-label follow-up studies suggested the same might be true in humans (Cui et al. 2001). Studies also suggested that lithium might increase clearance of marijuana metabolites through its strong diuretic properties and effects on fat metabolism (given that lipophilic THC lingers in fatty tissues) (Bergamaschi et al. 2013).

In a double-blind, placebo-controlled trial, 38 participants with marijuana dependence were admitted for 8 days to an inpatient withdrawal unit and were randomly assigned to receive either lithium carbonate (500 mg twice daily) or placebo (Johnston et al. 2014). Both groups received typical inpatient programming around relapse prevention. Follow-up interviews were conducted at intervals of 14, 30, and 90 days after discharge from the program. The lithium-treated group did not have lower overall withdrawal scores, but they did have reduced symptoms of loss of appetite, stomachaches, and nightmares or strange dreams. Lithium had no appreciable effects on either plasma oxytocin levels or on elimination of marijuana metabolites. Both the treatment and the placebo groups demonstrated reduction in the level of marijuana use and improved psychosocial outcomes 30 and 90 days after discharge, although there were no differences between the groups.

Although the clinical trial of lithium, which would putatively act by increasing oxytocin to ameliorate withdrawal symptoms, was negative, the result did not appear to be because of a failure of oxytocin pathways, as oxytocin levels were not increased. In laboratory studies, intranasal administration of oxytocin showed some promise in decreasing cravings and anxiety symptoms during withdrawal from marijuana (McRae-Clark et al. 2013).

Glutamate Modulators

N-acetylcysteine.   N-acetylcysteine (NAC) is an inexpensive, over-the-counter supplement that modulates glutamate activity and may be efficacious across a variety of psychiatric conditions. Specific effects on the cysteine-glutamate exchanger in the nucleus accumbens may correct a drug-induced pathology and may reduce drug-seeking behaviors.

In an 8-week double-blind, placebo-controlled study of marijuana-dependent adolescents and young adults, 116 participants were randomly assigned to receive either NAC 1,200 mg or placebo twice daily (Gray et al. 2012). Participants also took part in a robust CM intervention and brief weekly cessation counseling. Those in the NAC treatment group were more than twice as likely to submit urine drug screens negative for marijuana throughout the course of the study. At the final treatment visit, 40.9% of the urine drug screens in the NAC treatment group were negative for marijuana, compared with 27.2% in the placebo group. At the posttreatment follow-up visit, 19.0% of the urine drug screens in the NAC treatment group were negative for marijuana, compared with 10.3% in the placebo group. There were no significant differences between the groups in the occurrence of adverse events. Seventy of the 116 participants (60%) were retained through treatment completion, and 47% were retained through the posttreatment follow-up, with no significant differences in retention at either time point in the treatment or placebo groups. Via CM, participants in the NAC treatment group earned on average $162 for adherence and $86 for abstinence, and the placebo group earned an average of $141 for adherence and $54 for abstinence.

Future Directions

The literature exploring the use of medication-assisted treatments for problematic marijuana use and addiction has not yet reached maturity, and translational and laboratory research will continue to inform potential pharmacotherapeutic interventions to be used in conjunction with psychosocial interventions (Balter et al. 2014). The currently available literature suggests that there may be future roles for gabapentin and N-acetylcysteine for reducing withdrawal symptoms and promoting abstinence from marijuana. Currently, a large multisite randomized, placebo-controlled study of NAC for marijuana cessation in adults (Achieving Cannabis Cessation: Evaluating N-acetylcysteine Treatment; ACCENT) is being conducted via the National Drug Abuse Treatment Clinical Trials Network. Findings from further investigations of the role of gabapentin in managing withdrawal symptoms and promoting cessation are likely to be published in the near future as well. Preliminary data for each of these agents give reason to be cautiously optimistic.

Agonist therapies that target cannabinoid receptors may yet demonstrate clinical utility. Laboratory studies suggest that nabilone, a synthetic THC analogue approved by the FDA for the treatment of chemotherapy-induced nausea and vomiting, may have more potential as an agonist therapy than dronabinol, possibly because of better bioavailability and longer duration of action.

A novel drug target for the future may be one that increases endogenous cannabinoids rather than administering exogenous cannabinoids. Pharmacological agents that decrease the activity of the enzymes that degrade some endogenous cannabinoids—fatty acid amide hydrolase and monoacylglycerol lipase—have shown some promise in reducing marijuana withdrawal symptoms in mice.

Analogous to the use of the opioid receptor antagonist naltrexone in opioid use disorders, a cannabinoid type 1 (CB_1) receptor antagonist, rimonabant, showed some reduction in the acute effects of marijuana (Huestis et al. 2001), but psychiatric side effects have rendered it to be of unlikely benefit. Whether this is a class effect of CB_1 receptor antagonists, or whether other related agents could play a role, remains to be studied. Lofexidine, an α_2-adrenergic receptor agonist used in Europe to treat opioid withdrawal, has been shown to decrease gastrointestinal distress and improve sleep during withdrawal from marijuana in laboratory studies (Haney et al. 2008).

Summary

The developing literature on medication-assisted treatments for problematic marijuana use and addiction has thus far provided few clearly positive results. From the available data, there may be a role in the future for THC agonist therapies, and smaller clinical trials of gabapentin and NAC show promise, but these agents will require further investigation before definitive recommendations about their use in cannabis use disorders can be made.

The currently available studies of medication-assisted treatments for problematic marijuana use and addiction are generally underpowered to detect clinically significant effects and suffer from disturbingly high rates of dropout. Methodologies are heterogeneous in measuring marijuana withdrawal symptoms as well as abstinence or decreases in use.

Also contributing to possible failure to detect differences between pharmacological treatment arms is the fact that it is simply unethical to withhold the moderately effective psychosocial interventions from participants in clinical trials. Often, combinations of pharmacological and psychosocial interventions are superior to either intervention alone. Currently available psychopharmacological interventions do not appear to add much to psychosocial interventions, but that does not necessarily mean that the pharmacological intervention would not be more effective than placebo.

Antidepressants, buspirone, divalproex sodium, and lithium do not appear to be particularly useful for treating marijuana dependence per se, and little research informs a rational pharmacological approach to co-occurring psychiatric disorders with cannabis use disorder. Clinicians will unfortunately be left treating co-occurring disorders using separate pharmacological approaches.

Despite these limitations in the current literature, findings from basic science and human laboratory studies provide good reason for optimism that further clinical investigations may well yield clinically useful and possibly robust pharmacotherapeutic interventions for reducing the symptoms of marijuana withdrawal and promoting long-term abstinence.

Key Points

- Marijuana is the most commonly used illicit drug in the Western world. One in 10 adult marijuana users develops addiction, and the rates in adolescents are even higher. Significant misinformation about marijuana makes the treatment of marijuana addiction challenging.

- A treatment plan for problematic marijuana use and addiction starts with a thorough assessment of the reasons for, types of, and patterns of use while exploring motivation for change using the principles of motivational interviewing.
- The withdrawal syndrome following cessation of heavy marijuana use is real and is a significant barrier for individuals trying to stop using marijuana.
- Psychosocial interventions—including cognitive-behavioral therapy, relapse prevention, motivational enhancement therapy, and contingency management—are moderately effective for treating marijuana addiction.
- Although pharmacotherapy for marijuana withdrawal or addiction is an ongoing, active area of research, current data do not suggest a role for specific pharmacotherapy in the treatment of marijuana withdrawal or marijuana addiction. Preliminary data for cannabinoid agonists, gabapentin, and *N*-acetylcysteine suggest that continued investigation may reveal a more specific role for pharmacotherapy in the treatment of marijuana addiction in the future.

References

Allsop DJ, Copeland J, Lintzeris N, et al: Nabiximols as an agonist replacement therapy during cannabis withdrawal: a randomized clinical trial. JAMA Psychiatry 71(3):281–291, 2014 24430917

American Psychiatric Association: Diagnostic and Statistical Manual of Mental Disorders, 5th Edition. Arlington, VA, American Psychiatric Association, 2013

Babson KA, Ramo DE, Baldini L, et al: Mobile app-delivered cognitive behavioral therapy for insomnia: feasibility and initial efficacy among veterans with cannabis use disorders. JMIR Res Protoc 4(3):e87, 2015 26187404

Balter RE, Cooper ZD, Haney M: Novel pharmacologic approaches to treating cannabis use disorder. Curr Addict Rep 1(2):137–143, 2014 24955304

Bashford J, Flett R, Copeland J: The Cannabis Use Problems Identification Test (CUPIT): development, reliability, concurrent and predictive validity among adolescents and adults. Addiction 105(4):615–625, 2010 20403014

Benishek LA, Dugosh KL, Kirby KC, et al: Prize-based contingency management for the treatment of substance abusers: a meta-analysis. Addiction 109(9):1426–1436, 2014 24750232

Bergamaschi MM, Karschner EL, Goodwin RS, et al: Impact of prolonged cannabinoid excretion in chronic daily cannabis smokers' blood on per se drugged driving laws. Clin Chem 59(3):519–526, 2013 23449702

Budney AJ, Roffman R, Stephens RS, et al: Marijuana dependence and its treatment. Addict Sci Clin Pract 4(1):4–16, 2007 18292704

Budney AJ, Stanger C, Tilford JM, et al: Computer-assisted behavioral therapy and contingency management for cannabis use disorder. Psychol Addict Behav 29(3):501–511, 2015

Carpenter KM, McDowell D, Brooks DJ, et al: A preliminary trial: double-blind comparison of nefazodone, bupropion-SR, and placebo in the treatment of cannabis dependence. Am J Addict 18(1):53–64, 2009 19219666

Carroll KM, Easton CJ, Nich C, et al: The use of contingency management and motivational/skills-building therapy to treat young adults with marijuana dependence. J Consult Clin Psychol 74(5):955–966, 2006 17032099

Cornelius JR, Salloum IM, Ehler JG, et al: Fluoxetine in depressed alcoholics: a double-blind, placebo-controlled trial. Arch Gen Psychiatry 54(8):700–705, 1997 9283504

Cornelius JR, Salloum IM, Haskett RF, et al: Fluoxetine versus placebo for the marijuana use of depressed alcoholics. Addict Behav 24(1):111–114, 1999 10189977

Copeland J, Swift W, Roffman R, Stephens R: A randomized controlled trial of brief cognitive-behavioral interventions for cannabis use disorder. J Subst Abuse Treat 21(2):55–64, 2001 11551733

Copeland J, Gilmour S, Gates P, Swift W: The Cannabis Problems Questionnaire: factor structure, reliability, and validity. Drug Alcohol Depend 80(3):313–319, 2005 15916867

Cornelius JR, Bukstein OG, Douaihy AB, et al: Double-blind fluoxetine trial in comorbid MDD-CUD youth and young adults. Drug Alcohol Depend 112(1–2):39–45, 2010 20576364

Cui SS, Bowen RC, Gu GB, et al: Prevention of cannabinoid withdrawal syndrome by lithium: involvement of oxytocinergic neuronal activation. J Neurosci 21(24):9867–9876, 2001 11739594

Davis ML, Powers MB, Handelsman P, et al: Behavioral therapies for treatment-seeking cannabis users: a meta-analysis of randomized controlled trials. Eval Health Prof 38(1):94–114, 2015 24695072

Dennis M, Godley SH, Diamond G, et al: The Cannabis Youth Treatment (CYT) Study: main findings from two randomized trials. J Subst Abuse Treat 27(3):197–213, 2004 15501373

Diamond G, Panichelli-Mindel SM, Shera D, et al: Psychiatric syndromes in adolescents with marijuana abuse and dependency in outpatient treatment. J Child Adolesc Subst Abuse 15(4):37–54, 2006

Gates PJ, Norberg MM, Copeland J, et al: Randomized controlled trial of a novel cannabis use intervention delivered by telephone. Addiction 107(12):2149–2158, 2012 22632139

Ghaemi SN, Katzow JJ, Desai SP, et al: Gabapentin treatment of mood disorders: a preliminary study. J Clin Psychiatry 59(8):426–429, 1998 9721823

Gossop M, Darke S, Griffiths P, et al: The Severity of Dependence Scale (SDS): psychometric properties of the SDS in English and Australian samples of heroin, cocaine and amphetamine users. Addiction 90(5):607–614, 1995 7795497

Gray KM, Carpenter MJ, Baker NL, et al: A double-blind randomized controlled trial of N-acetylcysteine in cannabis-dependent adolescents. Am J Psychiatry 169(8):805–812, 2012 22706327

Hall W, Pacula RL: Cannabis Use and Dependence: Public Health and Public Policy. Cambridge, UK, Cambridge University Press, 2003

Haney M, Hart CL, Vosburg SK, et al: Effects of THC and lofexidine in a human laboratory model of marijuana withdrawal and relapse. Psychopharmacology (Berl) 197(1):157–168, 2008 18161012

Hoch E, Noack R, Henker J, et al: Efficacy of a targeted cognitive-behavioral treatment program for cannabis use disorders (CANDIS). Eur Neuropsychopharmacol 22(4):267–280, 2012 21865014

Huestis MA, Gorelick DA, Heishman SJ, et al: Blockade of effects of smoked marijuana by the CB1-selective cannabinoid receptor antagonist SR141716. Arch Gen Psychiatry 58(4):322–328, 2001 11296091

Johnston J, Lintzeris N, Allsop DJ, et al: Lithium carbonate in the management of cannabis withdrawal: a randomized placebo-controlled trial in an inpatient setting. Psychopharmacology (Berl) 231(24):4623–4636, 2014 24880749

Kadden RM, Litt MD, Kabela-Cormier E, Petry NM: Abstinence rates following behavioral treatments for marijuana dependence. Addict Behav 32(6):1220–1236, 2007 16996224

Karam-Hage M, Brower KJ: Gabapentin treatment for insomnia associated with alcohol dependence. Am J Psychiatry 157(1):151, 2000 10618048

Levin FR, McDowell D, Evans SM, et al: Pharmacotherapy for marijuana dependence: a double-blind, placebo-controlled pilot study of divalproex sodium. Am J Addict 13(1):21–32, 2004 14766435

Levin FR, Mariani JJ, Brooks DJ, et al: Dronabinol for the treatment of cannabis dependence: a randomized, double-blind, placebo-controlled trial. Drug Alcohol Depend 116(1–3):142–150, 2011 21310551

Levin FR, Mariani J, Brooks DJ, et al: A randomized double-blind, placebo-controlled trial of venlafaxine-extended release for co-occurring cannabis dependence and depressive disorders. Addiction 108(6):1084–1094, 2013 23297841

Lussier JP, Heil SH, Mongeon JA, et al: A meta-analysis of voucher-based reinforcement therapy for substance use disorders. Addiction 101(2):192–203, 2006 16445548

Marijuana Treatment Project Research Group: Brief treatments for cannabis dependence: findings from a randomized multisite trial. J Consult Clin Psychol 72(3):455–466, 2004 15279529

Marlatt GA, Donovan DM: Relapse Prevention: Maintenance Strategies in the Treatment of Addictive Behaviors, 2nd Edition. New York, Guilford, 2005

Martin G, Copeland J: The adolescent cannabis check-up: randomized trial of a brief intervention for young cannabis users. J Subst Abuse Treat 34(4):407–414, 2008 17869051

Mason BJ, Light JM, Williams LD, et al: Proof-of-concept human laboratory study for protracted abstinence in alcohol dependence: effects of gabapentin. Addict Biol 14(1):73–83, 2009 18855801

Mason BJ, Crean R, Goodell V, et al: A proof-of-concept randomized controlled study of gabapentin: effects on cannabis use, withdrawal and executive function deficits in cannabis-dependent adults. Neuropsychopharmacology 37(7):1689–1698, 2012 22373942

McHugh RK, Hearon BA, Otto MW: Cognitive behavioral therapy for substance use disorders. Psychiatr Clin North Am 33(3):511–525, 2010 20599130

McRae AL, Brady KT, Carter RE: Buspirone for treatment of marijuana dependence: a pilot study. Am J Addict 15(5):404, 2006 16966201

McRae-Clark AL, Carter RE, Killeen TK, et al: A placebo-controlled trial of buspirone for the treatment of marijuana dependence. Drug Alcohol Depend 105(1–2):132–138, 2009 19699593

McRae-Clark AL, Carter RE, Killeen TK, et al: A placebo-controlled trial of atomoxetine in marijuana-dependent individuals with attention deficit hyperactivity disorder. Am J Addict 19(6):481–489, 2010 20958842

McRae-Clark AL, Baker NL, Maria MM, et al: Effect of oxytocin on craving and stress response in marijuana-dependent individuals: a pilot study. Psychopharmacology (Berl) 228(4):623–631, 2013 23564179

Miller WR, Rollnick S: Motivational Interviewing, 3rd Edition. New York, Guilford, 2013

Penetar DM, Looby AR, Ryan ET, et al: Bupropion reduces some of the symptoms of marihuana withdrawal in chronic marihuana users: a pilot study. Subst Abus 6:63–71, 2012 22879754

Petry NM, Peirce JM, Stitzer ML, et al: Effect of prize-based incentives on outcomes in stimulant abusers in outpatient psychosocial treatment programs: a National Drug Abuse Treatment Clinical Trials Network study. Arch Gen Psychiatry 62(10):1148–1156, 2005 16203960

Rooke S, Copeland J, Norberg M, et al: Effectiveness of a self-guided Web-based cannabis treatment program: randomized controlled trial. J Med Internet Res 15(2):e26, 2013 23470329

Salinsky MC, Storzbach D, Spencer DC, et al: Effects of topiramate and gabapentin on cognitive abilities in healthy volunteers. Neurology 64(5):792–798, 2005 15753411

Stanger C, Ryan SR, Scherer EA, et al: Clinic- and home-based contingency management plus parent training for adolescent cannabis use disorders. J Am Acad Child Adolesc Psychiatry 54(6):445–453.e2, 2015 26004659

Stephens RS, Roffman RA, Simpson EE: Treating adult marijuana dependence: a test of the relapse prevention model. J Consult Clin Psychol 62(1):92–99, 1994 8034835

Stephens RS, Roffman RA, Curtin L: Comparison of extended versus brief treatments for marijuana use. J Consult Clin Psychol 68(5):898–908, 2000 11068976

Vandrey R, Smith MT, McCann UD, et al: Sleep disturbance and the effects of extended-release zolpidem during cannabis withdrawal. Drug Alcohol Depend 117(1):38–44, 2011 21296508

Weinstein AM, Miller H, Bluvstein I, et al: Treatment of cannabis dependence using escitalopram in combination with cognitive-behavior therapy: a double-blind placebo-controlled study. Am J Drug Alcohol Abuse 40(1):16–22, 2014 24359507

CHAPTER 9

Prevention of Marijuana Misuse

School-, Family-, and Community-Based Approaches

W. Alex Mason, Ph.D.

Charles B. Fleming, M.A.

Kevin P. Haggerty, Ph.D., M.S.W.

Clinical Vignette: Ryan at Templeton Middle School

Dr. Kimberly Stevens is a school psychologist at Templeton Middle School, a public school located in a low-income urban neighborhood of a mid-sized city in the midwestern United States. At the request of Ms. Ruth Hansen, an eighth-grade math teacher, Dr. Stevens has an appointment with Ryan Wilson, a 13-year-old student who recently moved to the area. Ms. Hansen indicated being concerned about how Ryan is handling the transition to a new school. He gets average grades and is generally well behaved, but occasionally he is disrespectful to Ms. Hansen and acts out in class. He has been slow to make friends but has recently been hanging out with Dennis Bailey and James Pierce, two classmates who are often tardy and struggle in school.

The writing of this chapter was supported in part by a grant from the National Institute on Drug Abuse (3R01DA025651). The content is solely the responsibility of the authors and does not necessarily represent the official views of the funding agency or the National Institutes of Health.

James was recently suspended for bringing marijuana to school. There are reports that a small number of students at the middle school smoke marijuana frequently, and it is known that marijuana is easily available to students at the local high school and in the neighborhood surrounding it.

Ryan sits in Dr. Stevens's office with arms folded. He says that he does not know why he has to see the school psychologist. Initially, his comments are short and abrupt, but he gradually warms up to Dr. Stevens and becomes talkative. Ryan reports that his father recently lost his job and moved the family into the city to find work but has not found anything yet. His parents are close in general, but they often argue about money. Ryan knows that his parents care about him, but he prefers to stay in his room or hang out with his new friends these days. He indicates that he sometimes feels like he does not fit in with others in school, but he has been getting to know Dennis and James and enjoys spending time with them. When asked what he would like to do with his life, Ryan says that he would like to go to college and make a lot of money but also says he is worried about high school because he knows the workload and pressures will be much greater and he has never been a great student.

Reflecting on her discussion with Ryan, Dr. Stevens concludes that he is a thoughtful boy who is struggling with a difficult relocation. She worries that he might get further off track and that his academic performance might suffer. She knows Ryan faces some struggles with family life at home, but she is comforted by the knowledge that his family seems close, aside from tensions and arguments about money. Dr. Stevens is concerned that Ryan has selected friends who have gotten in trouble and are involved in drugs and that peer influences might affect his transition to high school and, ultimately, his future. She has seen a number of students who become early marijuana and alcohol users, are labeled as "stoners," and struggle to finish high school. She is familiar with other school districts' drug use prevention programs, but her own school has not yet implemented one to benefit Ryan and other students.

Ryan may be at a turning point. His development as a teenager might take a bad path, leading to school difficulties, drug abuse, and related problems. Alternatively, he could take a more positive path, leading to school success and the avoidance of marijuana and other drug use. What factors in his life increase his risk for problematic marijuana use? What factors could protect him from such use? How can we intervene to help Ryan thrive and avoid the adverse consequences of drug involvement, including marijuana use? What prevention techniques are available and offer the most promise for Ryan and young people like him? These questions prompt us to consider how we can prevent the emergence of problems and promote positive development, rather than waiting until Ryan experiences problems that demand intervention.

Introduction: A Primer on Prevention

Problematic marijuana use and addiction, once established, are difficult and costly to treat. Fortunately, evidence suggests that marijuana use is preventable, although additional research and practice advancements are needed. Preventive interventions can have multiple goals. With respect to marijuana involvement, a primary goal may be to prevent the initiation of use and, therefore, to promote abstinence. Another goal of preventive intervention may be to reduce heavy use among marijuana use initiators. Yet another prevention-oriented goal may be to reduce the likelihood that individuals will experience harms, such as family and legal problems, resulting from marijuana use. All of these goals are legitimate and have a place in the development of a comprehensive strategy for preventing problematic marijuana use and addiction.

Programs that accomplish the multiple goals of prevention are grounded in longitudinal research that identifies risk and protective factors for a targeted outcome, such as marijuana use. Risk factors increase and protective factors decrease the likelihood of the outcome. Risk and protective factors optimally can be identified well before the adverse outcome develops, and many are malleable in the sense that they can be changed through intervention activities. Thus, hallmarks of prevention are early identification of risk and protective factors, followed by early intervention, most commonly among children, to decrease risk and increase protection before problems emerge and become deeply rooted (Coie et al. 1993). Prevention science recognizes that children develop under the influences of multiple socializing agents. Primary socializing influences on children are found within the school, the family, and the community domains. Accordingly, longitudinal research has identified risk and protective factors for marijuana use that fall within these domains (Substance Abuse and Mental Health Services Administration 2014). Table 9–1 illustrates selected school, family, and community risk and protective factors for marijuana use, as well as individual and peer risk and protective factors that cut across socializing domains.

On this foundation, effective substance use preventive interventions have been developed for implementation within the school, family, and community environments. Within each environment, preventive interventions may be universal or targeted (National Research Council and Institute of Medicine 2009). Universal preventive interventions are provided to all individuals who meet certain global criteria regardless of level of risk, such as all students in a school in grades 6–8. By contrast, targeted preventive interventions are directed toward at-risk individuals. One type of targeted intervention, *selective preventive intervention,* is provided to individuals who have risk factors that increase the likelihood that they will experience the targeted problem outcome. For example, adolescents of parents diagnosed with cannabis use disorder are at elevated risk for problematic marijuana use due to hereditary and environmental influences and could be targeted for selective preventive interventions to prevent the onset of marijuana use. Another type

TABLE 9–1. Selected risk and protective factors for adolescent marijuana use in the school, family, community, individual, and peer domains

	School	Family	Community	Individual	Peer
Risk factors	Poor grades	Higher family income	Community norms	Male gender	Peer drug use
	Truancy	Family conflict	Drug availability	Alcohol use	Peer delinquency
	Student drug use	Inconsistent discipline	Community crime	Cigarette use	
		Poor parenting	Community poverty	Conduct disorder	
		Parental drug use		Depression	
				Impulsivity	
				Intentions to use	
Protective factors	School rules	Household rules	Community laws	Perceived drug harms	Peer positive behavior
	School performance	Parental monitoring	Community policing	School achievement	
		Family involvement	Social embeddedness	Religiosity	
		Parent-child bonding			

TABLE 9–2.   The SAFE acronym for effective preventive interventions

Sequenced	Definition: A defined set of activities organized in a step-by-step fashion
	Example: Having a program manual that outlines learning objectives and steps
Active	Definition: An interactive format that encourages participant engagement
	Example: Providing role-play opportunities with feedback
Focused	Definition: An emphasis on social skills development
	Example: Training in problem solving and coping skills
Explicit	Definition: A targeted focus on content related to the outcome
	Example: Training in skills for refusing an offer to use marijuana

of targeted intervention, *indicated preventive intervention,* is provided to individuals who display early indicators of the targeted problem outcome. For example, middle school students who have initiated marijuana use could be targeted for indicated preventive interventions to prevent escalation of use and the development of marijuana-related problems.

Effective school-, family-, and community-based preventive interventions, whether they target marijuana use or other adverse outcomes, have been shown to share in common certain general characteristics, which likely contribute to their success (e.g., Gottfredson and Wilson 2003). As depicted in Table 9–2, these characteristics can be organized into an acronym: SAFE (Durlak et al. 2011). As described in more detail in the table, effective preventive interventions tend to be Sequenced, Active, Focused on social skills, and Explicit in targeting outcomes of interest. Research reviewed in this chapter suggests that preventive interventions that adopt these characteristics can help promote the positive development of youth. Such interventions also can provide economic benefits (Washington State Institute for Public Policy 2014). In this way, investments in effective prevention can pay off in the form of averted costs associated with problematic marijuana use and other adverse outcomes.

In this chapter we review the evidence base for youth problematic marijuana use prevention strategies. In subsequent sections, we briefly describe the legal and historical changes and basic scientific advancements that provide the backdrop for current marijuana use prevention research and practice. Next, we review evidence-based programs in the school, family, and community domains that have demonstrated, within the context of rigorous trials, significant effects on marijuana-related outcomes among youth. Drawing from themes across multiple studies, we outline some lessons learned to date and note areas where further research is needed to more fully realize the potential to effectively prevent problematic marijuana use. Finally, we conclude with policy and practice recommendations.

Legal, Historical, and Scientific Context of Marijuana Use Prevention Efforts

The legal status of marijuana in the United States has changed dramatically during the past two decades. At the time of this writing, 23 states and the District of Columbia had legalized some form of medical marijuana under varying degrees of regulation. Four states (Colorado, Washington, Oregon, and Alaska) and the District of Columbia had legalized recreational marijuana for adults age 21 years or older. Attitudes toward marijuana have also changed dramatically, with a slight majority (52%) of the U.S. public now supporting marijuana legalization according to the 2014 General Social Survey (Smith et al. 2015). Likewise, total marijuana consumption has risen among adults (Caulkins et al. 2015). Prevalence of marijuana use among adolescents, however, seems to have increased only slightly in recent years, following a period of declining use since the mid-1990s. For example, Monitoring the Future (MTF; Johnston et al. 2014) has been providing nationwide survey data on high school students since the 1970s. Marijuana use questions included in the MTF survey are illustrated in Table 9–3. Analyses of trends in MTF data found that the prevalence of past-month marijuana use among tenth graders was 20.5% in 1996, dropped steadily to 13.8% in 2008, rebounded to 18.0% in 2013, and then dropped slightly to 16.6% in 2014 (Johnston et al. 2014). The fluctuation in marijuana use prevalence over the past two decades contrasts with the long-term decline in cigarette smoking over the past 30 years as well as the steady decline in alcohol use over the past 15 years (Johnston et al. 2014). Furthermore, there are reasons to expect increases in adolescent marijuana use as the legal status of marijuana continues to evolve and new laws are implemented. In particular, legalization is likely to result in substantial reduction in the price of marijuana as well as increases in availability, factors that have been shown to play a role in the use of other drugs, such as alcohol, among young people (Wagenaar et al. 2010).

The potential for prevalence of adolescent marijuana use to increase in the coming years is a concern. Although research on the effects of occasional

---

TABLE 9–3. **Marijuana use questions included in the Monitoring the Future study**

On how many occasions (if any) have you used marijuana (weed, pot) or hashish (hash, hash oil)...

a. ...in your lifetime?

b. ...during the last 12 months?

c. ...during the last 30 days?

❑   0 occasions

❑   1–2 occasions

❑   3–5 occasions

❑   6–9 occasions

❑   10–19 occasions

❑   20–39 occasions

❑   40 or more

Source. Johnston et al. 2014.

marijuana use has not produced strong evidence of severe consequences (Pardini et al. 2015), the harmful effects of regular, heavy use of marijuana are well documented (Hall 2015; Volkow et al. 2014). Marijuana is generally considered to be less addictive than tobacco and does not have strong associations with violence and accidents, as does alcohol. However, 1 in 10 who try marijuana develop dependence symptoms (Hall 2015), and regular or heavy use in adolescence has been tied to long-term negative consequences. A review of research on long-term associations suggests that regular use doubles the risk of cognitive impairment and psychosis in adulthood (Hall 2015). Perhaps most disconcertingly, regular marijuana use among adolescents has a strong association with poor academic outcomes (Bachman et al. 2008). Although the causal mechanism is not clear, a review of studies found that regular marijuana use approximately doubles the chances of school dropout (Hall 2015).

Prevention of Problematic Marijuana Use and Addiction

Several reviews of youth substance use preventive interventions have been conducted (Hansen 1992; Tobler and Stratton 1997), and a few recent reviews that restrict their focus to marijuana use prevention are now available

(Faggiano et al. 2008; Norberg et al. 2013; Porath-Waller et al. 2010). Our goal in this section is not to duplicate those resources but to summarize conclusions drawn from previous work and briefly review programs and practices in each domain (school, family, and community) that have shown some evidence of effects on marijuana use outcomes, including onset, frequency, and quantity of use.

Prior to addressing each domain, it is important to note that prevention programs designed solely to address marijuana use are rare. Most of the field's successes in making an impact on marijuana-related outcomes have occurred within the context of general substance use prevention programs. Such programs either target substance use, broadly speaking, or include components related to the three most common types of substance use among adolescents in the United States: alcohol, tobacco, and marijuana (Johnston et al. 2014). Moreover, strictly individual-level programs are fairly rare in substance use prevention. Instead, as noted, youth substance use prevention programs tend to address individuals within one or more primary socialization contexts. Thus, individual, as well as peer-focused, components usually are incorporated into the curricula of school-, family-, and community-based prevention programs.

School-Based Prevention Strategies

School-based marijuana and other substance use prevention programs have received the greatest amount of attention from researchers and practitioners (Faggiano et al. 2008; Hansen 1992; Porath-Waller et al. 2010; Tobler and Stratton 1997). These programs have been classified as being either skills based or informational. Guided by social learning theories (Bandura 1977), skills-based programs typically focus on youth situated within the context of their social relationships (e.g., with teachers, classmates) and teach skills related to coping and problem solving, anger management, and conflict resolution, as well as peer substance use refusal techniques. Such programs tend to be interactive and place a premium on having youth practice new skills while also receiving support and guided feedback. Informational programs, on the other hand, emphasize increasing children's knowledge about drug use, including their understanding of the potential harms of using drugs. Both skills-based and informational programs often include components designed to limit youths' opportunity to use drugs—for example, by encouraging their involvement in prosocial activities, such as after-school sports, or increasing supervision by teachers and other adults. School-based programs vary in length, with some lasting as long as 3–5 years. Most such programs are implemented by teachers, but some use nonteachers (e.g., peers) as facilitators.

Independent research studies and meta-analyses have shown some evidence that school-based substance use prevention programs can be effective in preventing marijuana use initiation and reducing the frequency and quantity of marijuana use among youth, with small to medium effect sizes. For example, in their meta-analysis, Porath-Waller et al. (2010) reported a statistically significant mean weighted effect size of 0.58 across 15 studies for the impact of school-based substance use preventive interventions on reducing marijuana use among youth, which is medium in size. In another meta-analysis, Faggiano et al. (2008) reported that school-based programs resulted in a statistically significant reduction in marijuana use of about 20%. Studies have shown that interactive, skills-based school programs have stronger effects on marijuana use than didactic programs, which typically are informational (Faggiano et al. 2008). Moreover, programs that use nonteacher facilitators, such as peers, have been shown to have stronger effects than those that rely strictly on teachers, perhaps by capitalizing on peer influence processes during adolescence (Gottfredson and Wilson 2003). Studies on program length are mixed (Gottfredson and Wilson 2003; Norberg et al. 2013), although there is some evidence that longer programs (e.g., more than 15 sessions) and programs that include booster sessions can have stronger effects than shorter programs and those without boosters (Porath-Waller et al. 2010). Somewhat counterintuitively, effective prevention programs do not appear to need content that is specific to marijuana use to have an impact on this outcome; as noted previously, many effective school-based programs target substance use in general.

One of the most heavily researched and widely disseminated school-based substance use prevention programs is Drug Abuse Resistance Education (D.A.R.E.), which predominantly has been informational in scope. Although the program has been shown to have short-term effects on drug-related knowledge and attitudes, rigorous evaluations have not provided much support for D.A.R.E. as an effective program for preventing and reducing marijuana use, especially over the long term (e.g., Lynam et al. 1999).

Life Skills Training (LST) is a widely used school-based program that has shown some evidence of effects on marijuana-related outcomes as well other types of substance use (Botvin et al. 1990; Spoth et al. 2002). Effects of LST on marijuana use sometimes have been observed only for certain groups (e.g., those receiving a high dosage of the program) (Botvin et al. 1995) or under certain analysis conditions (e.g., in analyses that do not account for the clustering of students within schools) (Botvin et al. 2000, 2001). Grounded in social influence theories, LST seeks to prevent alcohol, tobacco, and marijuana use by reducing risks (e.g., negative peer influences) and promoting youth social competence (e.g., problem-solving skills). The middle school program serves students in grades 6–9 and is implemented as a sequence of classes and booster sessions over 3 years. Sessions focus on the development of self-management (e.g., problem solving), social (e.g., communication, assertiveness), and substance use refusal skills through instruction, modeling, and practice. In a series of studies, the developers of LST have pointed to evidence of effects on frequency of smoking marijuana (Botvin et al. 1990, 2000, 2001), particularly among students exposed to programs with a high degree of fidelity (Botvin et al. 1995). Significant effects on reduced marijuana initiation also were reported in an independent evaluation (Spoth et al. 2002). On the basis of these studies, which have also reported evidence of intervention effects on alcohol and tobacco use, LST currently is the most well-documented school-based substance use prevention program available. The Midwestern Prevention Project (also known as Project STAR) has as its central component a social learning–based school intervention for the prevention of substance use among middle school students. The program has had mixed effects on marijuana-related outcomes, with some indication of reduced past-month and past-week marijuana use (Johnson et al. 1990; Pentz et al. 1989), particularly under conditions of high implementation fidelity (Pentz et al. 1990).

Schools are natural places to gain access to a large number of children and adolescents. As such, they provide a venue in which to implement prevention programming with a large reach. Of course, there are some downsides to school-based preventive interventions. For example, youth who are highly mobile or who drop out of school are unlikely to receive the full program. Moreover, as the academic expectations placed on school districts are raised, there is decreasing time for activities perceived as falling outside the scope of the educational mandate. Teachers, in particular, have little time to implement prevention programming in the classroom. That being said, the promise of these types of programs is clear. School-based substance use preventive intervention currently represents the most well-documented strategy for preventing youth marijuana use. These programs are being used in schools throughout the country, although there is room for improvement in dissemination efforts. In one national survey, 35% of elementary schools reported using at least one school-based substance use prevention program, most commonly LST (24% of schools) (Hanley et al. 2010).

Family-Based Prevention Strategies

Second only to school-based strategies, family-based strategies for the prevention and reduction of marijuana and other substance use have received considerable attention (Velleman et al. 2005). These strategies are based on the premise that the family represents an early and enduring socializing influence on children, and they are grounded in fundamental theories of parent-child interaction patterns (Patterson 1982) as well as parenting styles (Baumrind 1967). Family-based substance use prevention programs typically target parents of early adolescents, timed prior to the onset of substance use for most youth. These programs generally are interactive and skills-based, including both general and substance-specific content. Skills development for parents focuses on communicating clear rules and guidelines for positive youth behavior, monitoring and supervising youth, and providing appropriate consequences and rewards for negative and positive behavior. Applied to marijuana use, for example, family-based prevention programs teach parents how to develop and communicate household rules that promote abstinence from marijuana use, or at least delay initiation until legal age in a growing number of states with legalized recreational marijuana use. Parents also are taught how to monitor their adolescents, being cognizant of the friends with whom they are spending time and being aware of the warning signs of drug involvement. When behavior is consistent with established rules, parents are encouraged to praise their adolescents in the form of positive attention and increased privileges. In the face of rule violations, parents are instructed to provide moderate and consistent discipline, typically in the form of lost or restricted privileges.

Family-based substance use prevention strategies also nearly always include the active involvement of youth. Similar to school-based programs, family-based programs teach youth basic skills related to social interactions, coping, problem solving, and anger management. Youth also are taught substance use refusal skills to help them reject drug offers from friends and acquaintances while redirecting maladaptive opportunities in the form of drug use into prosocial opportunities, such as participating in sports or other positive extracurricular activities. Finally, these programs also encourage positive parent-child involvement. Sometimes, families are encouraged to plan and participate in fun family activities, such as going to the park or watching a television show together. Parents usually are taught how to hold an effective family meeting, which is the forum in which discussions about drug use can take place. Ultimately, these programs can help parents and their adolescents develop closer ties within the context of warm and supportive relationships designed to facilitate healthy youth development (Kumpfer and Alvarado 2003).

As is the case for school-based programs, family-based programs rarely include a sole focus on marijuana use prevention and often include no content that is specific to marijuana (Velleman et al. 2005). These programs tend to be relatively brief, ranging from as few as 4 weekly sessions to as many as 15 or more sessions. There is considerable variety to the format of these programs. Commonly, family-based substance use prevention programs adopt a group workshop format, in which parents and their children meet together with other families at a convenient location within the community (e.g., school library, church). Other family-based programs are implemented by a trained facilitator with families in their homes. Less common are self-administered interventions that provide booklets or similar materials and allow families to progress at their own pace (Haggerty et al. 2007), often with some type of external support (e.g., by a phone facilitator).

Research studies have provided some support for the efficacy of family-based programs in preventing and reducing increases in substance use that would otherwise be seen (Foxcroft et al. 2003; Velleman et al. 2005), including marijuana use. However, average effects are small to moderate in size, which is consistent with the tendency for these programs to be brief and universal in focus. Some of the same basic principles documented for school-based prevention strategies have been found to hold true in family-based strategies. Interactive, skills-development programs for families tend to have stronger effects on marijuana and other substance use than those that are more didactic. Moreover, programs do not need to have dedicated marijuana-specific modules to impact marijuana use. Modules that address substance use in general appear to have relevance for marijuana-specific outcomes. Still, effective family-based prevention programs typically have demonstrated effects on the incidence, prevalence, and frequency of marijuana use; effects on higher-end patterns of marijuana use, such as heavy and problematic use or cannabis use disorders, have not been documented.

Two family-based substance use prevention programs are the Strengthening Families Program: For Parents and Youth 10–14 (SFP 10–14; formerly the Iowa Strengthening Families Program) and Guiding Good Choices (GGC; formerly the Preparing for the Drug Free Years program). SFP 10–14 is a seven-session, family-based prevention program for parents and youth. Each session is 2 hours in length. Parents and youth participate in separate, concurrent sessions in the first hour and join together in the second hour. Program components address family-related risk factors, such as family conflict and harsh discipline, as well as protective factors, such as parent-child bonding and parental monitoring. Parents and youth also learn and practice coping, problem-solving, and anger management skills. GGC is a five-session, family-based substance use prevention program. Parents attend four of the five sessions alone and work on skills related to promoting parent-child bonding by increasing opportunities for positive youth involvement in the family, helping adolescents develop skills for positive family involvement (e.g., participation in family governance), and learning how to reward positive behaviors and give appropriate discipline for negative behaviors. Adolescents attend with their parents in one of the sessions, which provides an opportunity for direct youth skills training related to coping, problem-solving, anger management, and substance use refusal skills.

SFP 10–14 and GGC were evaluated in a longitudinal, randomized controlled trial of rural families, comparing each intervention to a minimal contact control condition in which participants received general parenting newsletters. Both programs were shown to reduce the proportion of new marijuana users relative to the control condition out to 4 years past baseline assessment, although only at a trend level for GGC (Spoth et al. 2001). Neither SFP 10–14 nor GGC has demonstrated strong effects on the frequency of marijuana use, although significant effects on reduced initiation and frequency of alcohol and cigarette use have been reported consistently, with effects lasting throughout adolescence and even into early adulthood (Spoth et al. 2009). It is noteworthy that the primary test of SFP 10–14 and GGC has been conducted among predominantly white participants in rural Iowa, which leaves unanswered questions about the potential generalizability of findings. Additional studies are needed.

As a primary socializing influence on children, the family represents a natural target for preventive interventions. Parenting and family interaction patterns are strong predictors of marijuana and other substance use (see Table 9–1). Thus, addressing risk and protective factors in the family is a strategy that holds considerable promise for preventing marijuana use, as demonstrated in tests of such programs as SFP 10–14. Of course, there are limitations to family-based substance use preventive interventions. In particular, several studies have documented low family engagement rates. For example, Spoth et al. (2007a) reported engagement rates in a large-scale implementation of family-based preventive interventions ranging from 11.2% to 30.8% (16.9% on average). Thus, a large proportion of targeted participants are not being reached by these programs. Families are often stressed and overburdened, and it is difficult for parents and their children to find the time to complete a prevention program. For workshop-based programs provided in the community, transportation and child care concerns are common. Innovations are being developed to address these challenges. For example, many programs are incorporating the principles and practices of motivational interviewing to increase participants' buy-in and active engagement in the program. In addition, self-administered programs allow participants to engage with program materials at their own convenience in their own homes (Haggerty et al. 2007). Family-based programs have garnered support with regard to preventing marijuana initiation, and rapidly developing innovations likely will enhance existing effects associated with this important class of prevention programming.

Community-Based Prevention Strategies

Community-based marijuana and other substance use prevention strategies are multifaceted and, overall, have received less systematic attention than school- and family-based programs. Such strategies include laws that prohibit marijuana use (e.g., among minors in states that have legalized recreational marijuana use for adults age 21 years and older). Another community-based prevention approach involves the use of public service announcements (PSAs) to discourage marijuana use among youth (Palmgreen et al. 2001). For example, in both Colorado and Washington State, radio and television PSAs have been developed and circulated to inform residents about what is legal and illegal under the new recreational marijuana laws (e.g., driving under the influence of marijuana is illegal). Another type of community prevention strategy adopts a place-based systems approach. Typically, this approach involves community-wide assessment of needs, followed by the selection and targeted implementation of evidence-based school- and family-based prevention programs. For example, a community needs assessment might reveal that rates of marijuana use are elevated among youth in a particular area. In this case, collaborative community partnerships would be formed involving government officials, school personnel, and community members to support the implementation of substance use prevention programs, such as LST and SFP 10–14, that have demonstrated effects on marijuana use. As illustrated in Figure 9–1, place-based prevention systems are designed to lead to the implementation of evidence-based substance use prevention programs on a wide scale through community coalitions and working groups. This approach is hypothesized to decrease risk factors and increase protective factors in the community, ultimately leading to the prevention of substance use and the promotion of positive behavior among youth (Brown et al. 2011).

Systematic reviews of the effects of community-based prevention strategies on marijuana use outcomes are lacking. However, independent studies of various community-based prevention strategies have produced promising results. For example, Sensation Seeking Targeting (SENTAR) is a prevention approach that targets marijuana use among high-sensation-seeking adolescents through televised anti-marijuana campaigns (Palmgreen et al. 2001). Campaigns primarily provide information about the risks related to marijuana use, including adverse effects on relationships and health (e.g., lung damage). A controlled evaluation of the media campaigns was conducted in three counties in the southeastern United States. Results showed that the intervention was associated with reductions in past-30-day marijuana use among high-sensation-seeking adolescents during a developmental period in which marijuana use typically increases among such youth. Campaign effects were specific to marijuana use and, in one county, persisted for several months after the television ads were taken off the air. Research on the SENTAR approach provides evidence that media campaigns can have their intended effects by reducing marijuana use among high-risk adolescents.

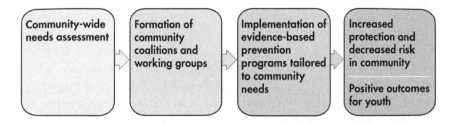

FIGURE 9–1. The place-based community prevention strategy: a general logic model.
Source. Adapted from Brown et al. 2011.

PROmoting School-community-university Partnerships to Enhance Resilience (PROSPER) and Communities That Care (CTC) are place-based intervention systems that seek to prevent substance use and other problems at a population level through the implementation of evidence-based prevention programs in a particular community setting. Briefly, PROSPER capitalizes on the land-grant university Cooperative Extension System to promote state-, university-, and community-level partnerships designed to facilitate the selection and implementation of proven family-based (e.g., SFP 10–14) and school-based (e.g., LST) preventive interventions. A large-scale, community-randomized trial of PROSPER demonstrated positive intervention effects on a number of targeted outcomes, including reduced marijuana initiation and past-year frequency of marijuana use among youth in intervention communities compared with those in control communities, with effects lasting 18 months and 4½ years past baseline (e.g., Spoth et al. 2007b). CTC is a widely disseminated community-based intervention system that trains communities to organize coalitions of diverse stakeholders to rally around the goal of preventing adolescent drug use and delinquency. Communities are trained to conduct a needs assessment and then select from a list of evidence-based preventive interventions those programs that best match their unique needs (see Figure 9–1). CTC provides training and supports to ensure that selected programs are implemented with fidelity and outcomes are monitored. A large-scale, community-randomized trial of CTC has not demonstrated effects on marijuana use. The trial found some evidence of positive effects of CTC on related behaviors, including reductions in the initiation and frequency of alcohol and tobacco use in early adolescence in a cohort of participants followed longitudinally from the outset of the study (Hawkins et al. 2009), although those effects were not maintained later in adolescence (Hawkins et al. 2014).

Youth are situated within and influenced by their surrounding communities. Community-level risk factors for marijuana use include factors such as the ready availability of marijuana and norms favorable to marijuana use (see Table 9–1). Intervening to reduce risk factors and increase protective factors at this level may be a potent prevention strategy. Moreover, community intervention provides an opportunity to reach youth at a population level. Media campaigns and place-based prevention systems, such as PROSPER and CTC, are designed to saturate a targeted area with evidence-based prevention programming, with the goal of improving public health by reducing substance use, delinquency, and related problem behaviors among large numbers of youth. These are ambitious, large-scale approaches. They can be costly and require considerable investment of time and effort on the part of community members (e.g., to help diffuse prevention messages or to be an active member of a community prevention coalition). Still, community-based prevention approaches are garnering some positive evidence to support their success, and additional advancements hold promise for preventing and reducing adolescent marijuana use on a wide scale.

Additional Marijuana Use Prevention Settings and Strategies

Most marijuana and other substance use prevention research has focused on school-, family-, and community-based programs, as reviewed previously, but alternatives do exist. Clinic-based substance use prevention programs are relatively rare, with the exception of brief alcohol interventions designed to prevent problematic alcohol use and addiction among college students and relapse prevention efforts (Dimeff et al. 1999), which represent more specialized types of prevention for higher-risk individuals. Partly guided by provisions of the Affordable Care Act, significant strides are being made in more fully integrating prevention into primary care settings, such as pediatric clinics. Project Chill brief interventions are universal prevention programs for adolescents (ages 12–18 years) who have not initiated marijuana use. These interventions are delivered in the context of urban federally qualified health centers and include either a therapist-delivered program or a self-administered, computer-based program. Both programs emphasize motivational interviewing principles, role-play scenarios, and role-modeling of positive behavior in risky settings (e.g., in the face of a drug offer). Evaluation results showed that the therapist-delivered program reduced certain risks associated with marijuana use (e.g., delinquency). Effects on marijuana use outcomes were restricted to the computer-based program, which was effective in preventing marijuana use initiation, as well as reducing the frequency of marijuana use among youth who started using during the follow-up period (Walton et al. 2014).

There is a growing body of research on self-administered substance use prevention programs (e.g., Haggerty et al. 2007), which have the advantage of allowing targeted participants to work through materials at their own pace, anytime and anywhere. This flexibility can increase participant engagement in the program and maximize intervention dosage. Project Chill is an example of one particularly valuable intervention delivery approach: self-administration via computer. Schinke et al. (2004) tested the efficacy of a substance use prevention program for early adolescents (ages 10–12) delivered via CD-ROM to reduce increases in marijuana use that occur in the broader population, as well as other substance use. The program, which is based on social learning theory, includes components related to coping and problem solving, effective communication, and substance use refusal skills. Results showed that the frequency of past-month marijuana use was lower among youth assigned to the CD-ROM program condition compared with youth in the control condition. Prevention research is rapidly incorporating the latest developments in information technology to reach and engage a wider audience. As many such studies are just getting under way, it is not clear what impact digital preventive interventions, such as Web-based or social media–driven programs, will have on marijuana-related outcomes, but the promise is considerable.

It is important to note that designations of preventive interventions as school, family, community, or clinic based can be artificial. Although some prevention programs do fall neatly into one of these categories, many cut across categories. For example, it is not uncommon for school-based substance use prevention programs to include some type of parenting component. Community-based prevention approaches often implement school- and/or family-based programming. Indeed, the most effective prevention programs incorporate multiple components across domains. Tiered prevention strategies represent one particularly valuable multicomponent approach. These strategies systematically integrate universal and targeted prevention programming. For example, the Family Check-Up (FCU) is a tiered family-focused intervention model delivered in middle schools. The FCU includes a universal prevention component in the form of a family resource center, which is located in the school setting and is staffed by a trained parent consultant. The parent consultant offers all families in the school general information and services related to student behavior and academics as well as parent training. At a more targeted level, the FCU model is also designed to identify at-risk students, who are referred to more intensive services. Specifically, the FCU offers a three-session, family-based intervention for at-risk students and their families. These sessions are based on motivational interviewing principles and include an assessment of family strengths and needs. Families then are provided with a menu of intervention services, including parent training, school-based intervention, and community resources that are tailored to their unique needs. If required, additional referrals also are offered to families. Evaluations of the FCU have produced positive results on a number of targeted outcomes, including substance use. In one test, results showed that the FCU led to improvements in student self-regulation (i.e., effortful control), a proximal target of the program, and that these improvements led, in turn, to reductions in the frequency of marijuana use over grades 6–8 (Fosco et al. 2013). Marijuana and other substance use are multidetermined behaviors, and it stands to reason that effective prevention strategies must address multiple risk and protective factors across individual, school, family, and community domains.

Principles of Effective Marijuana Use Prevention Strategies

As reflected in this chapter, research has identified principles that underlie many effective substance use prevention strategies. These principles are summarized in Figure 9–2 and can be nested within the broader characteristics of effective programs as represented by the SAFE acronym. Again, this acronym highlights that effective substance use prevention programs tend to be Sequenced, Active, Focused on skills, and Explicit in targeting substance use outcomes (see Table 9–2). Substance use prevention programs with significant effects on marijuana use tend to be grounded in social learning theory and provide participants with instruction in new attitudes and activities, examples or models of desired behaviors, and opportunities to practice new skills with immediate and constructive feedback (e.g., role-play scenarios). Skills practice is the best way to ensure that participants internalize what they have learned and increases the likelihood that new skills will be implemented in real-world interactions beyond the classroom or workshop. Thus, rather than relying heavily on didactic methods, effective substance use prevention programs are interactive and encourage the active involvement of participants. Because participant attendance and engagement in prevention programming are challenging, effective interventions often include motivational interviewing components to promote participants' readiness and willingness to change.

A common theme across the interventions reviewed here is that effective marijuana use prevention programs are skills based. Such skills include those related to social interactions (e.g., communication), effective problem solving (e.g., avoiding impulsive reactions), and coping with adversity in adaptive (e.g., relying on positive supports) rather than maladaptive (e.g., turning to marijuana use) ways. Substance use–specific information and

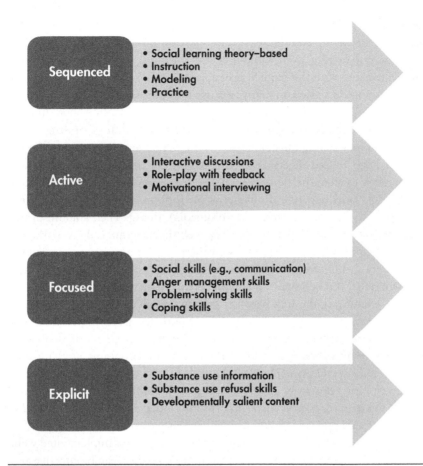

FIGURE 9–2. Principles of effective marijuana and other substance use prevention programs.

skills development activities also are common. Effective substance use prevention programs include developmentally salient information about substance use patterns and norms and commonly include skills development for youth related to refusing a drug offer from a friend or acquaintance (e.g., being passed a joint at a party).

Interestingly, research reviews suggest that substance use prevention programs do not need to have marijuana-specific components to have an impact on marijuana use outcomes. Risk factors for marijuana use are shared in common with other types of substance use, as well as many other non-substance-related problem behaviors (e.g., delinquency), among adolescents. For instance, family conflict in the home, lack of parental monitoring, and internalizing symptoms (e.g., depression) can increase risk for marijuana as well as alcohol and tobacco use. Thus, an alcohol use prevention program, for example, might have an impact on marijuana use by reducing common risk factors, even without ever mentioning marijuana. That being said, consistent with the Explicit principle of the SAFE acronym, preventive intervention effect sizes on marijuana use outcomes might be larger if programs include marijuana-specific content, such as information about unique adverse consequences of marijuana intake compared with other drugs.

Even the best programs grounded in the principles illustrated in Figure 9–2 will have limited effects if they are not implemented properly. *Implementation* refers to all of the elements of delivering a program. Dane and Schneider (1998) outlined five dimensions of implementation: fidelity (i.e., adherence to the manual and other protocols), dosage (i.e., amount of the intervention received), quality (i.e., how well the program is delivered), participant responsiveness (i.e., how well the program engages participants), and program differentiation (i.e., what makes a program unique). Durlak and DuPre (2008) conducted a comprehensive review of the prevention literature, examining the link between program implementation and impact. They found strong support for the conclusion that good implementation leads to better outcomes. Effect sizes for effective programs implemented well were two to three times larger than those for programs implemented poorly. This general principle likely holds for the specific case of marijuana use prevention (Botvin et al. 1995; Pentz et al. 1990), although additional studies are needed. Norberg et al. (2013) noted that reporting of implementation has been poor in studies of marijuana use prevention to date.

When guided by the above-mentioned principles and implemented well, marijuana and other substance use prevention strategies can be effective and cost-beneficial. The Washington State Institute for Public Policy (2014) recently reviewed prevention programs with some evidence of effects on marijuana use outcomes among youth, evaluating the costs and benefits of each program. Results suggested that prevention programs with effects on marijuana use and other outcomes can be a wise investment. For example, the institute reported that for LST, one of the evidence-based programs included in the review, every dollar invested in the program may provide an estimated return of $35.66. Given the serious and costly adverse consequences associated with marijuana use, even modest success in preventing those consequences can reap significant societal benefits and cost savings.

Next Steps in Research and Practice

Significant advancements have been made in the science and practice of marijuana use prevention, although important gaps remain and further work is needed. Effects of many effective school-, family-, and community-based programs on marijuana use outcomes have been small to medium in size and sometimes last only for a short duration. Moreover, few substance use prevention programs have demonstrated effects on indicators of problematic marijuana use, such as heavy use and addiction. These comments are not to imply that small intervention effect sizes on marijuana initiation and related outcomes are trivial. Indeed, an intervention with a modest effect size in preventing marijuana initiation, when implemented on a large scale to a wide audience, can have a significant impact on improved public health by reducing the incidence of marijuana use in a targeted population. Still, effect sizes of substance use preventive interventions on marijuana-related outcomes might be improved with strategic program adaptations.

As mentioned, effect sizes on marijuana use might be improved by incorporating marijuana-specific components into general substance use preventive interventions. Such components could include psychoeducational content about the epidemiological patterns and the consequences of adolescent marijuana use, as well as skills development focused, for example, on parental monitoring of marijuana use (e.g., recognizing marijuana paraphernalia and the signs of being high on marijuana) and adolescent refusal of offers to use marijuana. In the changing climate of marijuana legalization, these types of adaptations may be essential. It is unknown if existing evidence-based substance use prevention programs will have effects on marijuana use outcomes in the context of legalized recreational marijuana use. There is a strong need for tests of existing substance use prevention programs, likely with some adaptations, within the context of marijuana legalization, as well as for the development and evaluation of new preventive interventions tailored for the changing legal climate.

An important debate in research and practice concerns the tension between fidelity of program delivery and adaptation. Notwithstanding evidence that high program fidelity leads to better outcomes, there often is room for adaptation. Indeed, as noted by Durlak and DuPre (2008), program adaptations sometimes can improve outcomes by helping providers tailor programming to the needs of targeted schools, families, communities, and youth. Durlak and DuPre (2008) advocate for striking the proper balance between program fidelity, particularly adherence to the core components and essential principles of effective interventions, and adaptation. Adaptations of substance use preventive interventions for the context of marijuana legalization will need to consider this balance. Of course, more significant adaptations call for new evaluations using rigorous methods to test whether the intended effects on marijuana-related outcomes are achieved.

Unfortunately, few evidence-based programs with demonstrated effects on marijuana use are being implemented on a wide scale for public health benefit. This science-to-practice gap has generated a new frontier of research designed to understand what it takes to disseminate and implement evidence-based preventive interventions on a large scale. Too many programs benefit participants only within the context of the randomized trials in which those programs are being evaluated. More thought needs to be given at the early stages of program development and evaluation to the matter of how to ensure that programs will be adopted by service providers and used to attain broad reach within the targeted population of participants. Again, this might require strategic program adaptations. For example, a marijuana use prevention program for youth may lack cultural sensitivity. In this case, adaptations, guided by research methods that place a premium on incorporating the valued perspectives of targeted participants, could be made to enhance the cultural relevance and desirability of the program. Ultimately, effective marijuana use prevention programs will need to be implemented widely to achieve maximum impact in communities throughout the United States.

Policy and Practice Recommendations

Although further research is needed to enhance our understanding of how to prevent problematic marijuana use and addiction, it is not too early to act on existing knowledge. We conclude this chapter with specific recommendations for policymakers and for practitioners interested in implementing marijuana use prevention strategies.

At a policy level, there should be a significant investment in evidence-based prevention. Currently, the Substance Abuse and Mental Health Services Administration (SAMHSA) provides block grants to states to support substance abuse prevention services. Expanded funding opportunities would be valuable. This is particularly true in light of the changing U.S. landscape regarding the legalization of marijuana. Prevention approaches at all levels—family, school, and community—are needed to help promote the positive development of our nation's youth by avoiding the potential adverse consequences of marijuana use. As reviewed previously, research shows that funds spent on the implementation of evidence-based preventive interventions are a good investment, providing short- and long-term benefits to society.

Our strongest recommendation for practitioners is to use available evidence-based prevention programs with demonstrated effects from rigorous trials on marijuana use outcomes among youth. The most well-supported programs are school based (e.g., LST), and it is known that school programs can play a critical role in a comprehensive prevention strategy for promoting the positive development of youth on a large scale. Across school, family, and community domains, readers are encouraged to seek out available review articles and meta-analyses that detail evidence-based programs (Faggiano et al. 2008; Foxcroft et al. 2003; Norberg et al. 2013; Porath-Waller et al. 2010; Velleman et al. 2005). Moreover, online resources are available in the form of evidence-based program registries, such as Blueprints for Healthy Youth Development (www.blueprintsprograms.com/), the National Registry of Evidence-based Programs and Practices (NREPP; www.samhsa.gov/nrepp), and the California Evidence-Based Clearinghouse for Child Welfare (CEBC; www.cebc4cw.org/). These registries provide searchable databases that can be used to identify evidence-based prevention programs that have had an impact on marijuana use and other outcomes. In addition to information about the programs themselves (e.g., components, training requirements), these registries provide information about the quality of evaluation studies to allow practitioners to direct their attention to the most well-supported programs in their areas of interest (Gandhi et al. 2007).

There are, of course, circumstances in which it will not be feasible to use an existing evidence-based program—for example, because of funding or other practical constraints. Likewise, until more research is completed, the extent to which newly developed or significantly adapted prevention programs have desired effects on targeted outcomes remains unknown. It can take several years for evidence in support of a program to accrue, and failing to take action when needed can be undesirable and even unethical. Under these circumstances, practitioners who must move forward with implementing a marijuana use prevention strategy are encouraged to use evidence-supported principles and practices, such as those listed in Figure 9–2. In particular, it is known that marijuana and other substance use prevention programs should be interactive and skills based; simply providing knowledge (e.g., about the adverse effects of drugs) is not enough. Using evidence-supported principles and practices increases the likelihood that intervention activities will lead to intended outcomes. Still, the best way to ensure that intervention efforts will be effective in preventing and reducing marijuana use is to implement one or more evidence-based programs with documented effects on marijuana outcomes.

Key Points

- Longitudinal research has identified school, family, community, individual, and peer risk and protective factors for adolescent marijuana and other substance use. Substance use prevention programs seek to reduce risk factors and enhance protective factors in youth.

- Substance use prevention programs have been developed primarily for implementation in three socialization contexts: school, family, and community. Marijuana-specific programs are rare; most programs address substance use in general.
- School-based substance use prevention programs have been the most well-researched. Systematic reviews and meta-analyses report that school-based programs can reduce marijuana use among youth at small to medium effect sizes. Currently, the Life Skills Training (LST) program has received the most research support.
- Both family- and community-based preventive interventions have shown some evidence of effectiveness in reducing the rate of marijuana initiation among youth, although effect sizes have been small and effects sometimes have been short in duration.
- Individual-level substance use prevention programs have been rare, to date, although clinic-based and self-administered interventions do exist. There is some evidence that these programs are effective in reducing the frequency of marijuana use among youth, but more research is needed.
- Research has begun to identify characteristics and principles of effective substance use prevention programs. In particular, such programs tend to be Sequenced, Active, Focused on skills development, and Explicit in targeting substance-related knowledge and skills (SAFE).
- Although more research is needed, it is not too early to act on existing knowledge. Practitioners are encouraged to implement evidence-based substance use prevention programs, particularly in the school domain, and to adopt evidence-supported principles and practices.

References

Bachman JG, O'Malley PM, Schulenberg JE, et al: The Education-Drug Use Connection: How Successes and Failures in School Relate to Adolescent Smoking, Drinking, Drug Use, and Delinquency. New York, Taylor & Francis Group/Lawrence Erlbaum, 2008

Bandura A: Social Learning Theory. Englewood Cliffs, NJ, Prentice Hall, 1977

Baumrind D: Child care practices anteceding three patterns of preschool behavior. Genet Psychol Monogr 75(1):43–88, 1967 6032134

Botvin GJ, Baker E, Dusenbury L, et al: Preventing adolescent drug abuse through a multimodal cognitive-behavioral approach: results of a 3-year study. J Consult Clin Psychol 58(4):437–446, 1990 2212181

Botvin GJ, Baker E, Dusenbury L, et al: Long-term follow-up results of a randomized drug abuse prevention trial in a white middle-class population. JAMA 273(14):1106–1112, 1995 7707598

Botvin GJ, Griffin KW, Diaz T, et al: Preventing illicit drug use in adolescents: long-term follow-up data from a randomized control trial of a school population. Addict Behav 25(5):769–774, 2000 11023017

Botvin GJ, Griffin KW, Diaz T, et al: Drug abuse prevention among minority adolescents: posttest and one-year follow-up of a school-based preventive intervention. Prev Sci 2(1):1–13, 2001 11519371

Brown EC, Hawkins JD, Arthur MW, et al: Prevention service system transformation using Communities That Care. J Community Psychol 39(2):183–201, 2011 23606774

Caulkins JP, Kilmer B, Kleiman MAR, et al: Considering Marijuana Legalization: Insights for Vermont and Other Jurisdictions. Santa Monica, CA, RAND Corporation, 2015

Coie JD, Watt NF, West SG, et al: The science of prevention: a conceptual framework and some directions for a national research program. Am Psychol 48(10):1013–1022, 1993 8256874

Dane AV, Schneider BH: Program integrity in primary and early secondary prevention: are implementation effects out of control? Clin Psychol Rev 18(1):23–45, 1998 9455622

Dimeff LA, Baer JS, Kivlahan DR, et al: Brief Alcohol Screening and Intervention for College Students (BASICS): A Harm Reduction Approach. New York, Guilford, 1999

Durlak JA, DuPre EP: Implementation matters: a review of research on the influence of implementation on program outcomes and the factors affecting implementation. Am J Community Psychol 41(3–4):327–350, 2008 18322790

Durlak JA, Weissberg RP, Dymnicki AB, et al: The impact of enhancing students' social and emotional learning: a meta-analysis of school-based universal interventions. Child Dev 82(1):405–432, 2011 21291449

Faggiano F, Vigna-Taglianti FD, Versino E, et al: School-based prevention for illicit drugs use: a systematic review. Prev Med 46(5):385–396, 2008 18258289

Fosco GM, Frank JL, Stormshak EA, et al: Opening the "Black Box": Family Check-Up intervention effects on self-regulation that prevents growth in problem behavior and substance use. J Sch Psychol 51(4):455–468, 2013 23870441

Foxcroft DR, Ireland D, Lister-Sharp DJ, et al: Longer-term primary prevention for alcohol misuse in young people: a systematic review. Addiction 98(4):397–411, 2003 12653810

Gandhi AG, Murphy-Graham E, Petrosino A, et al: The devil is in the details: examining the evidence for "proven" school-based drug abuse prevention programs. Eval Rev 31(1):43–74, 2007 17259575

Gottfredson DC, Wilson DB: Characteristics of effective school-based substance abuse prevention. Prev Sci 4(1):27–38, 2003 12611417

Haggerty KP, Skinner ML, MacKenzie EP, et al: A randomized trial of Parents Who Care: effects on key outcomes at 24-month follow-up. Prev Sci 8(4):249–260, 2007 17987388

Hall W: What has research over the past two decades revealed about the adverse health effects of recreational cannabis use? Addiction 110(1):19–35, 2015 25287883

Hanley SM, Ringwalt C, Ennett ST, et al: The prevalence of evidence-based substance use prevention curricula in the nation's elementary schools. J Drug Educ 40(1):51–60, 2010 21038763

Hansen WB: School-based substance abuse prevention: a review of the state of the art in curriculum, 1980–1990. Health Educ Res 7(3):403–430, 1992 10171672

Hawkins JD, Oesterle S, Brown EC, et al: Results of a type 2 translational research trial to prevent adolescent drug use and delinquency: a test of Communities That Care. Arch Pediatr Adolesc Med 163(9):789–798, 2009 19736331

Hawkins JD, Oesterle S, Brown EC, et al: Youth problem behaviors 8 years after implementing the Communities That Care prevention system: a community-randomized trial. JAMA Pediatr 168(2):122–129, 2014 24322060

Johnson CA, Pentz MA, Weber MD, et al: Relative effectiveness of comprehensive community programming for drug abuse prevention with high-risk and low-risk adolescents. J Consult Clin Psychol 58(4):447–456, 1990 2212182

Johnston LD, O'Malley PM, Bachman JG, et al: Monitoring the Future National Survey Results on Drug Use, 1975–2013, Vol 1: Secondary School Students. Ann Arbor, Institute for Social Research, University of Michigan, 2014

Kumpfer KL, Alvarado R: Family-strengthening approaches for the prevention of youth problem behaviors. Am Psychol 58(6–7):457–465, 2003 12971192

Lynam DR, Milich R, Zimmerman R, et al: Project DARE: no effects at 10-year follow-up. J Consult Clin Psychol 67(4):590–593, 1999 10450631

National Research Council and Institute of Medicine: Preventing Mental, Emotional, and Behavioral Disorders Among Young People: Progress and Possibilities. Washington, DC, National Academies Press, 2009

Norberg MM, Kezelman S, Lim-Howe N: Primary prevention of cannabis use: a systematic review of randomized controlled trials. PLoS One 8(1):e53187, 2013 23326396

Palmgreen P, Donohew L, Lorch EP, et al: Television campaigns and adolescent marijuana use: tests of sensation seeking targeting. Am J Public Health 91(2):292–296, 2001 11211642

Pardini D, White HR, Xiong S, et al: Unfazed or dazed and confused: does early adolescent marijuana use cause sustained impairments in attention and academic functioning? J Abnorm Child Psychol 43(7):1203–1217, 2015 25862212

Patterson GR: Coercive Family Process. Eugene, OR, Castalia, 1982

Pentz MA, Dwyer JH, MacKinnon DP, et al: A multicommunity trial for primary prevention of adolescent drug abuse: effects on drug use prevalence. JAMA 261(22):3259–3266, 1989 2785610

Pentz MA, Trebow WB, Hansen WB, et al: Effects of program implementation on adolescent drug use behavior. Eval Rev 14(3):264–289, 1990

Porath-Waller AJ, Beasley E, Beirness DJ: A meta-analytic review of school-based prevention for cannabis use. Health Educ Behav 37(5):709–723, 2010 20522782

Schinke SP, Schwinn TM, Di Noia J, et al: Reducing the risks of alcohol use among urban youth: three-year effects of a computer-based intervention with and without parent involvement. J Stud Alcohol 65(4):443–449, 2004 15376818

Smith TW, Marsden PF, Hout M: General Social Surveys, 1972–2014. Chicago, IL, National Opinion Research Center, 2015

Spoth RL, Redmond C, Shin C: Randomized trial of brief family interventions for general populations: adolescent substance use outcomes 4 years following baseline. J Consult Clin Psychol 69(4):627–642, 2001 11550729

Spoth RL, Redmond C, Trudeau L, Shin C: Longitudinal substance initiation outcomes for a universal preventive intervention combining family and school programs. Psychol Addict Behav 16(2):129–134, 2002 12079251

Spoth R, Clair S, Greenberg M, et al: Toward dissemination of evidence-based family interventions: maintenance of community-based partnership recruitment results and associated factors. J Fam Psychol 21(2):137–146, 2007a 17605536

Spoth R, Redmond C, Shin C, et al: Substance-use outcomes at 18 months past baseline: the PROSPER Community-University Partnership Trial. Am J Prev Med 32(5):395–402, 2007b 17478265

Spoth R, Trudeau L, Guyll M, et al: Universal intervention effects on substance use among young adults mediated by delayed adolescent substance initiation. J Consult Clin Psychol 77(4):620–632, 2009 19634956

Substance Abuse and Mental Health Services Administration: Risk and Protective Factors Associated With Youth Marijuana Use: Using Prevention Research to Guide Prevention Practice (Ref #HHSS277200800004C). Washington, DC, Substance Abuse and Mental Health Administration, Center for the Application of Prevention Technologies, 2014

Tobler NS, Stratton HH: Effectiveness of school-based drug prevention programs: a meta-analysis of the research. J Prim Prev 18(1):71–128, 1997

Velleman RDB, Templeton LJ, Copello AG: The role of the family in preventing and intervening with substance use and misuse: a comprehensive review of family interventions, with a focus on young people. Drug Alcohol Rev 24(2):93–109, 2005 16076580

Volkow ND, Baler RD, Compton WM, et al: Adverse health effects of marijuana use. N Engl J Med 370(23):2219–2227, 2014 24897085

Wagenaar AC, Tobler AL, Komro KA: Effects of alcohol tax and price policies on morbidity and mortality: a systematic review. Am J Public Health 100(11):2270–2278, 2010 20864710

Walton MA, Resko S, Barry KL, et al: A randomized controlled trial testing the efficacy of a brief cannabis universal prevention program among adolescents in primary care. Addiction 109(5):786–797, 2014 24372937

Washington State Institute for Public Policy: Preventing and treating youth marijuana use: an updated review of the evidence. Olympia, Washington State Institute for Public Policy, 2014

Index

Page numbers printed in **boldface** type refer to boxes, figures, or tables.

ABCD (Adolescent Brain Cognitive Development) study, 7
ACCENT (Achieving Cannabis Cessation: Evaluating N-acetylcysteine Treatment), 193
ACE models of genetic and environmental risks used in twin studies, 23, **23**
Acetaminophen
  interactions with marijuana, **93**
Achieving Cannabis Cessation: Evaluating N-acetylcysteine Treatment (ACCENT), 193
Addiction, 17–21
  failed inhibition of craving and relapse to drug seeking, 19, **20**
  inhibition of craving, 19, **19**, 24, **25**
  initial intoxication and, 17, **18**
  marijuana dependence and withdrawal, 30–31, 32
  pharmacological dependence, 30–31
  repeated use of marijuana and, 17, **19**, 21
  treatment, 171–198
ADHD. See Attention-deficit/hyperactivity disorder
Adolescent Brain Cognitive Development (ABCD) study, 7
Adolescents
  adverse effects of marijuana use in, **91**
  brain development in, 21–22
  clinical vignette of marijuana use at age 13, 11–13
  developmental effects of marijuana use, 32, 144
  with marijuana addiction, 183

mesolimbic system of, 19–20
  prevalence of marijuana use in, 204–205
  risk and protective factors for marijuana use, 201, **202**
  use of marijuana, 5
Adolescent vulnerability hypothesis, 22
Adults and use of marijuana, 5–6
Advocacy groups, 5
Affordable Care Act, 214
AIDS
  indications for medical marijuana, 80–81
Alaska
  indications for medical marijuana program enrollment and levels of clinical evidence, **53**
  medical marijuana program passage and characteristics, **48**, 204
Alcohol
  interaction with marijuana, **93**
  marijuana use and, **103**
  onset of use, 24, **24**
  psychosis and, **122**
ALS. See Amyotrophic lateral sclerosis
Alzheimer's dementia, 86
Amotivational syndrome, 16
Amprenavir
  interactions with marijuana, **93**
Amyotrophic lateral sclerosis (ALS)
  indications for medical marijuana, 85–86
Anandamide, 8
Anesthetics
  interactions with marijuana, **93**

Anticoagulants
  interactions with marijuana, **93**
Anticonvulsants
  for treatment of marijuana addiction,
    190–192
Antidepressants
  for treatment of marijuana addiction,
    187–189
    norepinephrine reuptake inhibi-
      tors, 188
    selective serotonin reuptake
      inhibitors, 187
    serotonin-norepinephrine reup-
      take inhibitors, 188
Antiemetics, 83
Antifungals
  interactions with marijuana, **93**
Anxiety
  indications for medical marijuana,
    88–89
  marijuana comorbidity and, 107–109
  marijuana use and, **103**
  synthetic cannabinoids and, 158
Anxiety disorders, 107–108
  treatment of marijuana addiction
    and, 174
Anxiolytics
  psychosis and, **122**
  for treatment of marijuana addiction,
    190
2-Arachidonylglycerol, 8
Arizona
  indications for medical marijuana
    program enrollment and levels
    of clinical evidence, **53**
  medical marijuana program passage
    and characteristics, **48**
Army Substance Abuse Program, 154
Aromatherapy, 152
Ashworth scale, 82
Aspergillus, 3, 8, 73, 76, 78–79, 186
Atomoxetine
  for treatment of marijuana addiction,
    188

Attention-deficit/hyperactivity disor-
    der (ADHD)
  marijuana comorbidity and, 111–112
    case vignette of, 101–102
  marijuana use and, 12, **103**
Australia, 104, 139
Australian National Cannabis Preven-
    tion and Information Centre, 174
Austria, 157

Baltimore Epidemiologic Catchment
    Area study (1980), 109
Behavioral health conditions
  marijuana comorbidity and, 102,
    103
Benzoylindoles, **153**
Bipolar disorder, 107
  marijuana use and, **103**
  substance use disorder and, 27–28
"Black Diamond," 152, 159
"Black Mamba"
  case vignette of, 149–151
  logo for, **151**
Blueprints for Healthy Youth Develop-
    ment, 221
Brief psychotic disorder
  DSM-5 criteria for, **122–123**
Buspirone
  for treatment of marijuana addiction,
    190

Calcium channel blockers
  interactions with marijuana, **93**
California
  compassionate access initiative, 58
  indications for medical marijuana
    program enrollment and levels
    of clinical evidence, **53**
  legal protections for possession of
    marijuana for medicinal pur-
    poses, 46, **47**
  medical marijuana program passage
    and characteristics, **48**
  Proposition 215, **44**

California Evidence-Based Clearing-house for Child Welfare (CEBC), 221
CAMS (Cannabinoids in Multiple Sclerosis) study, 82
Canada
  approved use of nabiximols, 73
  medical marijuana use in, 57
Cannabichromene, 73
Cannabicyclohexanol, 154
Cannabidiol (CBD; Epidiolex), 3, **75**
  laws pertaining to, 59
Cannabigerol, 73
Cannabinodiol, 73
Cannabinoids, 3. *See also* Marijuana
  basics of, 73
  evidence for use of marijuana, 57
  formulations of marijuana, 76, **77**
    dispensary, 73, 76
    pharmaceutical, 73, **74–75**
  marijuana strains and varieties, 76
  synthetic, 64–65, 149–169
    clinical effects of, 158–161
      medical, 160–161, **160**
      psychiatric, 158–160, **159**
    clinical management of toxicity, misuse, and dependence on, 163–164
    clinical vignette of, 149–151
    development of, 152, **153**
    emergence of, 151–154
    epidemiology of use of, 154–157
    future directions for research on, 164–165
    legality of, 157–158
    versus marijuana, 161–163, **162**
    most commonly identified compounds, 152, **153**
  for treatment of marijuana addiction, 186–187
    dronabinol, 186
    nabiximols, 186–187
Cannabinoids in Multiple Sclerosis (CAMS) study, 82
Cannabinol, 73

Cannabis. *See also* Marijuana
  Cannabis indica, 76
  Cannabis sativa, 3, 8, 73, 76, 186
Cannabis-induced psychotic disorder, 12–13
Cannabis Problems Questionnaire, 174
Cannabis use disorder
  according to DSM-IV, 29
  according to DSM-5, 17, 21, 28
  prevalence and risks of, 21–31
    marijuana dependence and withdrawal, 30–31
    progression from marijuana use to addiction, 28–30
    risk factors for use of marijuana, 22–28, **23, 24, 25**
Cannabis Use Problems Identification Test (CUPIT), 174
Cannabis Youth Treatment Study, 183
Carter, Jimmy (President), 45
CB$_1$ receptor, 3, 8, 111, 137, 152, 166, 193–194
  activation of, 13–14
CB$_2$ receptor, 3, 137
CBD. *See* Cannabidiol
CBT. *See* Cognitive-behavioral therapy
CDC (Centers for Disease Control and Prevention), 155
CEBC (California Evidence-Based Clearinghouse for Child Welfare), 221
Center for Substance Abuse Treatment, 183
Centers for Disease Control and Prevention (CDC), 155
Central nervous system depressants
  interactions with marijuana, **93**
Cesamet. *See* Nabilone
Chemotherapy agents
  interactions with marijuana, **93**
Chlorzoxazone
  interactions with marijuana, **93**
Cimetidine
  interactions with marijuana, **93**
Cisapride
  interactions with marijuana, **93**

Clarithromycin
  interactions with marijuana, **93**
Clinical Global Impression–
  Improvement scale, 188
Clinical vignettes
  of marijuana use and comorbidity,
    101–102
  of marijuana use and mental health,
    1–2
  of marijuana use at age 13, 11–13
  for prescription of medical mari-
    juana, 39–40
  of prevention of marijuana misuse,
    199–200
  of psychotic disorder and marijuana
    use, 119–120
  of request for medical marijuana,
    71–72
  of synthetic cannabinoids, 149–151
  of treatment of marijuana addiction,
    171–172
Clopidogrel
  interactions with marijuana, **93**
CM. *See* Contingency management
Cocaine, 4, 41, 42, **43**, 104, 107, 111,
  113, **122**, 173, 180, 189
Cognition. *See* Neurocognition
Cognitive-behavioral therapy (CBT),
  178–179
Colorado
  Constitutional Amendment 64, 62
  indications for medical marijuana
    program enrollment and levels
    of clinical evidence, **53**
  legalization of recreational mari-
    juana, **44**
  medical marijuana program passage
    and characteristics, **48**, 204
Communities That Care (CTC), 213,
  214
Community-based prevention strategies, **202**, 211–214, **213**, 222
Comprehensive Drug Abuse Prevention and Control Act, 44–45, **43**

Conant v. Walters, 58
Conduct disorder
  treatment of marijuana addiction
    and, 174
Confounding hypothesis, 131
Connecticut
  indications for medical marijuana
    program enrollment and levels
    of clinical evidence, **53**
  legalization of medical marijuana,
    45–46
  medical marijuana program passage
    and characteristics, **48**
Constitutional Amendment 64 (Colorado), 62
Contingency management (CM)
  prize incentives contingency man-
    agement, 180
  for treatment of marijuana addiction,
    179–180
  voucher-based reinforcement, 180
Contraceptive drugs
  interactions with marijuana, **93**
Controlled Substances Act (CSA), 4, 6,
  43, 44–45, 59
Corticosteroids
  interactions with marijuana, **93**
Crohn's disease
  indications for medical marijuana, 85
CSA. *See* Controlled Substances Act
CTC (Communities That Care), 213,
  214
CUPIT (Cannabis Use Problems Identification Test), 174
Cyclohexylphenols, **153**
Cyclosporine
  interactions with marijuana, **93**

Dalteparin
  interactions with marijuana, **93**
D.A.R.E. (Drug Abuse Resistance Edu-
  cation), 207
DEA. *See* U.S. Drug Enforcement
  Administration

Delaware
 indications for medical marijuana
  program enrollment and levels
  of clinical evidence, **53**
 medical marijuana program passage
  and characteristics, **48**
Delay discounting, 28
Delta-8-tetrahydrocannabinol, 73
Delta-9-tetrahydrocannabinol (THC),
 2–3, 8, 152, 166, 174
 effects on developing brain, 11
 marijuana's psychoactive properties
  and, 73
 synthetic analogues to, 57
Dementia
 indications for medical marijuana, 86
Denmark, 143
Depression
 indications for medical marijuana, 88
 marijuana use and, **103**
 treatment of marijuana addiction
  and, 174
Derailment, 121
Development and marijuana's effects,
 31–32
Dialectical behavior therapy, 179
Dibenzo(b,d)pyrans, **74**
Diclofenac
 interactions with marijuana, **93**
Diltiazem
 interactions with marijuana, **93**
"Dime bag," 174–175
Dispensary formulations of marijuana,
 73, 76
Disulfiram
 interactions with marijuana, **93**
Divalproex sodium
 for treatment of marijuana addiction,
  190–191
Domestic Cannabis Eradication/Sup-
 pression Program, 2
Dopamine and marijuana use, 21
Dravet syndrome, 83
"Dream," 152

Dronabinol (Marinol), 73, **74,** 78, 80, 94
 for treatment of marijuana addiction,
  186
Drug Abuse Resistance Education
 (D.A.R.E.), 207
DSM-IV
 cannabis use disorder in, 29
DSM-5
 cannabis use disorder in, 17, 21, 28
 criteria for brief psychotic disorder,
  122–123
 criteria for cannabis withdrawal, 177,
  177
 criteria for schizophrenia, **124–126**
 criteria for schizophreniform disorder, **123–124**
 criteria for substance/medication-
  induced psychotic disorder,
  126–127
 posttraumatic stress disorder in, 27
Dysphoria, 130

Edibles, **77**
Efavirenz, 80
Endocannabinoid system, 3
Enflurane
 interactions with marijuana, **93**
Enoxaparin
 interactions with marijuana, **93**
Epidiolex. *See* Cannabidiol
Epilepsy, 83
Erythromycin
 interactions with marijuana, **93**
Estonia, 157
Estrogens/hormone therapy
 interactions with marijuana, **93**
Ethanol
 interactions with marijuana, **93**
Etiological hypothesis, 131
Etoposide
 interactions with marijuana, **93**
Euphoric recall, 20
European Monitoring Center for Drugs
 and Drug Addiction, 153–154

Families
  interventions for treatment of mari-
    juana addiction, 183
  prevention strategies for marijuana
    use, **202**, 208–211, 222
Family Check-Up (FCU), 215–216
FCU (Family Check-Up), 215–216
FDA. *See* U.S. Food and Drug Adminis-
    tration
Fexofenadine
  interactions with marijuana, **93**
Fluoxetine
  interactions with marijuana, **93**
France, 157

GABA$_A$ agonist, 190
GABAergic inhibitory neurons, 14
Gabapentin, 193
  for treatment of marijuana addiction,
    191
GAD. *See* Generalized anxiety disorder
Gateway hypothesis, 103, 106
  skepticism about, 106
Gender and marijuana's effects on
    development, 32
Generalized anxiety disorder (GAD),
    108, 109
  marijuana use and, **103**
General Social Survey, 204
Germany, 157
GGC (Guiding Good Choices), 210, 211
Glaucoma
  indications for medical marijuana, 84
Glutamate modulators
  for treatment of marijuana addiction,
    193
Gonzales v. Raich, **44**
Government. *See also* Legislation
  federally licensed marijuana cultiva-
    tion, **43**
  first medical marijuana program, **44**
  Ogden memo, **44**
  Shafer Commission Report, 45
  state legislation of recreational mar-
    ijuana, **44**

"Green Giant," 152
Guiding Good Choices (GGC), 210, 211

Hallucinations, 120–121
Hallucinogens
  psychosis and, **122**
Halothane
  interactions with marijuana, **93**
Harrison Narcotics Tax Act of 1914,
    42, **43**
Hashish, **77**
Hash oil, **77**
Hastening hypothesis, 138–139
Hawaii
  indications for medical marijuana
    program enrollment and levels
    of clinical evidence, **53**
  medical marijuana program passage
    and characteristics, **48**
HCV. *See* Hepatitis C virus
Health care utilization and marijuana
    use, 142
Health Related Behaviors Survey of
    Active Duly Military Personnel, 154
Heparin
  interactions with marijuana, **93**
Hepatitis C virus (HCV)
  indications for medical marijuana,
    84–85
Herbs, 152
Heroin, 6, 41, 103, 104, 173
Histamine H$_2$ antagonists
  interactions with marijuana, **93**
HIV
  indications for medical marijuana,
    80–81
Huffman, J.W., 152
HU synthetic cannabinoids, 152, **153**
Hypnotics
  psychosis and, **122**
  for treatment of marijuana addiction,
    190
Hypomania
  marijuana-medication interactions
    and, **93**

Ibuprofen
  interactions with marijuana, **93**
ICD-10
  cannabis withdrawal and, 31
Illicit drugs, 194–195
  marijuana use and, **103**, 105
Illinois
  indications for medical marijuana
    program enrollment and levels
    of clinical evidence, **54**
  medical marijuana program passage
    and characteristics, **48**
"Incense," 165
Indian warrior *(Pedicularis densiflora)*,
    152
Indinavir
  interactions with marijuana, **93**
Inhalants
  psychosis and, **122**
Institute of Regulation and Control of
    Cannabis (Uruguay), 64
Interaction hypothesis, 131
Intraocular pressure, 55, 84
Investigational drug permit, 59
Iowa Strengthening Families Program,
    210
Pedicularis densiflora (Indian warrior),
    152
IQ, 92
  developmental effects of marijuana
    use in adolescents, 32
  effects of marijuana use, 15
Isoflurane
  interactions with marijuana, **93**
Itraconazole
  interactions with marijuana, **93**

Jim Crow laws, 5
JWH compounds, 152, **153**

"K2," 150–151, **151**, 165
Ketoconazole
  interactions with marijuana, **93**
Kief, **77**
"Kronic," 151–152, 165

Lactation
  adverse effects of marijuana during,
    91–92
Lansoprazole, 80
Leary, Timothy, 44
Legislation. *See also* Government
  Affordable Care Act, 214
  Comprehensive Drug Abuse Pre-
    vention and Control Act, **43**,
    44–45
  Constitutional Amendment 64
    (Colorado), 62
  Controlled Substances Act, 4, 6, **43**,
    44–45, 59
  Harrison Narcotics Tax Act of 1914,
    42, **43**
  Jim Crow laws, 5
  laws pertaining to cannabidiol, 59
  marijuana laws by state, **47**
  Marijuana Tax Act of 1937, 42, **43**,
    44
  Misuse of Drugs Act of 1971
    (United Kingdom), 63
  ongoing, 6–7
  Proposition 215 (California), **44**
  Pure Food and Drug Act, **43**
  Safety and Innovation Act of 2012,
    64–65
  Synthetic Drug Abuse Prevention
    Act, 64–65, 157
Leonotis leonurus (wild dagga), 152
Life Skills Training (LST), 207–208, 222
Lithium
  for treatment of marijuana addiction,
    191–192
Lithuania, 157
Loose associations, 121
Loperamide
  interactions with marijuana, **93**
Louisiana
  legalization of medical marijuana,
    45–46
Lovastatin
  interactions with marijuana, **93**
LSD (lysergic acid diethylamide), 6

LST (Life Skills Training), 208, 222
Luxembourg, 157
Lysergic acid diethylamide (LSD), 6

Maine
    indications for medical marijuana
        program enrollment and levels
        of clinical evidence, **54**
    medical marijuana program pas-
        sage and characteristics, **48**
Major depressive disorder (MDD), 107,
    187
Mania
    indications for medical marijuana, 88
Marihuana. *See* Marijuana
Marijuana. *See also* Cannabinoids;
    Medical marijuana
    acute intoxication effects of, 13–14
    addiction, 17–21
        failed inhibition of craving and
            relapse to drug seeking, 19,
            20
        inhibition of craving, 19, **19**, 24,
            25
        initial intoxication, 17, **18**
        repeated use, 17, **19**, 21
    advocacy groups, 5
    beneficial versus detrimental effects
        of use of, 8
    biological factors and, 28–30
    classification as Schedule I substance,
        59
    coming-down phase of, 14, 16
    comorbidity and use of, 101–118
        anxiety, 107–109
        associated behavioral health
            problems, 102, **103**
        attention-deficit/hyperactivity
            disorder, 111–112
        clinical relevance of, 107, 110–111
        clinical vignette of, 101–102
        marijuana use as gateway to mari-
            juana use disorders, 106
        mood disorders, 108–110
        posttraumatic stress disorder, 111

        priming effect and, 107
        risk for substance use disorders,
            102–103, **104**
        risk for violence and suicide, 113
        sequential risk model and, 104–
            105
        skepticism about causal gateway
            progression, 106–107
        sleep disturbances, 112
        social determinants of mental
            health, 112
        risk, course, and outcomes of
            other psychiatric disorders,
            111–112
    dependence and withdrawal, 30–31
    directionality of marijuana-psychosis
        association, 131–132
    dopamine and, 21
    drug control policy, 40–42
    edibles, 175–176
    effects
        on development, 31–32
        on IQ, 15
        on the mind, 11–37
        on motivation, 16
    endocannabinoid system, 3
    euphoric effects of, 14
    extracts, 175
    history of policy, 42–45, **43–44**
    home cultivation of, 62
    medical policy of, 39–60
        marijuana laws by state, **47**
        medical programs, 46–59
            medical orientation, 46, 51–52
            participation in, 52, 57
        physician liability and, 59
        program passage and character-
            istics of, **44, 48–50**
        reimbursement and, 58
        symbolic reform of, 45–46
        Veterans Affairs and, 59–60
    medication interactions, 92, **93**
    mental health professionals and, 6–7
    neurocognition and, 15
    ongoing legislation of, 6–7

onset of use, 24, **24, 25**
overview, 1–9
plant, 2–3
  eradication of, 2
prevention of misuse of, 199–225
  clinical vignette of, 199–200
  indicated preventive intervention, 203
  legal, historical, and scientific context of, 204–205
  Monitoring the Future study, 204, **205**
  overview, 200–204
  policy and practice recommendations, 220–221
  prevention strategies
    community-based, 211–214, **213**
    family-based, 208–211
    school-based, 206–208
  principles of effective prevention strategies, 216–218, **217**
  research and practice, 218–220
  risk and protective factors for adolescent marijuana use, 201, **202**
  SAFE for effective prevention interventions, 203, **203**
  selective preventive intervention, 201
  use prevention settings and strategies, 214–216
price elasticity, 40–41
recreational policy of, 60–64
  case studies, 62
  decriminalization and commercial legalization of, 60–62
  international perspectives of, 62–64
risk factors for use of, 22–28, **23, 24, 25**
sale
  on black market, 61–62
  in commercial stores, 61
social constraints of, 30

synthetic cannabinoids, 64–65, 149–169
versus synthetic cannabinoids, 161–163, **162**
treatment of addiction to, 171–198
  assessment of marijuana use, 172–178
    assessment of amounts and types of marijuana use, 174–176
    motivations, triggers for use, and barriers to quitting, 176–177
    screening tools, 174
  clinical vignette of, 171–172
  pharmacological interventions, 185–194, 195
    anticonvulsants, 190–192
    antidepressants, 187–189
    anxiolytics, 190
    cannabinoids, 186–187
    future directions of, 193–194
    glutamate modulators, 193
    hypnotics, 190
    mood stabilizers, 190–192
  psychosocial interventions and motivational strategies, 178–185, 195
    cognitive-behavioral therapy, 178–179
    contingency management, 179–180
    effectiveness of, 181, **182**
    interventions with families, 183
    motivational enhancement therapy, 181, **182**
    relapse prevention, 178–179
    software-based technological interventions, 183–184
  trends in use of, 5–6
  in the United States, 4–7
  withdrawal from, 177–178
Marijuana Tax Act of 1937, 42, **43,** 44
Marinol. *See* Dronabinol

Marshmallow leaves, 152
Maryland
  medical marijuana program passage and characteristics, **48**
Massachusetts
  compassionate access initiative, 58
  indications for medical marijuana program enrollment and levels of clinical evidence, **54**
  medical marijuana program passage and characteristics, **49**
MDD (major depressive disorder), 107, 187
Medical marijuana, 6, 8, 71–99. *See also* Marijuana; Marijuana, medical policy of
  adverse effects of, 90–92, **91**
    marijuana-medication interactions, 92, **93**
    in pregnancy and lactation, 91–92
  cannabinoid basics and formulations of, 73–77
    additional formulations, 76, **77**
    basics of cannabinoids, 73
    dispensary formulations of marijuana, 73, 76
    marijuana strains and varieties, 76
    pharmaceutical formulations of marijuana, 73, **74–75**
  clinical vignette of request for, 71–72
  daily use of, 85
  DSM-5 criteria for substance/medication-induced psychotic disorder, **126–127**
  indications for use, 80–87
    amyotrophic lateral sclerosis, 85–86
    appetite enhancement in HIV/AIDS, 80–81
    Crohn's disease, 85
    dementia, 86
    glaucoma, 84
    hepatitis C, 84–85
    nausea, 83
    pain, 81–82

Parkinson's disease, 87
    seizures, 83–84
    spasticity and multiple sclerosis, 82–83
  metabolism and monitoring of, 78–80
    in the clinical setting, 79–80
    pharmacokinetics, 78, **79**
    quality control, 78–79
  psychiatric conditions and, 87–90
    anxiety, 88–89
    depression, 88
    mania, 88
    posttraumatic stress disorder, 89–90
    psychosis, 87–88
    sleep-wake disturbances, 90
Medical programs, 56–59
  medical orientation, 46, 51–52
  participation in, 52, 57
  program passage and characteristics of, **48–50**
Mental health
  clinical vignette of marijuana use and, 1–2
  psychiatric symptoms prior to marijuana use, 27
  social determinants of, 112
Mental health professionals
  assessment of patient needs, 32
  marijuana and, 6–7
  medical marijuana program awareness, 8
MET. *See* Motivational enhancement therapy
Metabolism
  in the clinical setting, 79–80
  monitoring of, 78–80
  pharmacokinetics and, 78, **79**
Methoxyflurane
  interactions with marijuana, **93**
MI. *See* Motivational interviewing
Michigan
  indications for medical marijuana program enrollment and levels of clinical evidence, **54**

medical marijuana program passage and characteristics, **49**
Midwestern Prevention Project, 208
Minnesota
    indications for medical marijuana program enrollment and levels of clinical evidence, **54**
    medical marijuana program passage and characteristics, **49**
Mississippi
    federally licensed marijuana cultivation, **43**
Misuse of Drugs Act of 1971 (United Kingdom), 63
Models
    for drug control policy, 41–42
    gateway hypothesis, 103, 106
    for marijuana legalization, 61
    reasoned action approach, 26
    sequential risk model for marijuana comorbidity, 104–105
    shared diathesis model, 139
    stepping stone theory, 103
    of temporal progression of drug use, 103, **104**
    theory of planned behavior, 26
Monitoring the Future (MTF) study, 16
    use questions, 204, **205**
Montana
    indications for medical marijuana program enrollment and levels of clinical evidence, **55**
    medical marijuana program passage and characteristics, **49**
Mood disorders
    marijuana comorbidity and, 108–110
Mood stabilizers
    for treatment of marijuana addiction, 190–192
Motivation and effects of marijuana use, 16
Motivational enhancement therapy (MET), **182**
Motivational interviewing (MI), 176–177
MS. *See* Multiple sclerosis

MTF. *See* Monitoring the Future study
Multiple sclerosis (MS)
    indications for medical marijuana, 82–83

Nabilone (Cesamet), 73, **74,** 78, 80, 94
Nabiximols (Sativex), 73, **75,** 82
    for treatment of marijuana addiction, 186–187
NAC. *See* N-acetylcysteine
N-acetylcysteine (NAC), 193
    for treatment of marijuana addiction, 192–193
Naproxen
    interactions with marijuana, **93**
National Comorbidity Survey, 108, 109
National Drug Abuse Treatment Clinical Trials Network, 193
National Epidemiologic Survey on Alcohol and Related Conditions (NESARC), 109
National Forensic Laboratory Information System (NFLIS), 157
National Institute on Drug Abuse, 7
National Institutes of Health, 7
National Longitudinal Survey of Youth, 109–110
National Poison Data System, 155
National Registry of Evidence-based Programs and Practices (NREPP), 221
Nausea
    indications for medical marijuana, 83
Nefazodone
    for treatment of marijuana addiction, 188–189
Nelfinavir
    interactions with marijuana, **93**
NESARC (National Epidemiologic Survey on Alcohol and Related Conditions), 109
The Netherlands, 63, 143
Neurocognition
    marijuana use and, 15, 32
    perception of time with marijuana use, 15

Nevada
  indications for medical marijuana
    program enrollment and levels
    of clinical evidence, **55**
  medical marijuana program passage
    and characteristics, **49**
New Hampshire
  indications for medical marijuana
    program enrollment and levels
    of clinical evidence, **55**
  legalization of medical marijuana,
    45–46
  medical marijuana program passage
    and characteristics, **49**
New Jersey
  indications for medical marijuana
    program enrollment and levels
    of clinical evidence, **55**
  Medicaid program in, 52
  medical marijuana program passage
    and characteristics, **49**
New Mexico
  indications for medical marijuana
    program enrollment and levels
    of clinical evidence, **55**
  medical marijuana program passage
    and characteristics, **49**
New York
  indications for medical marijuana
    program enrollment and levels
    of clinical evidence, **55**
  medical marijuana program passage
    and characteristics, **49**
New Zealand, 106, 113
NFLIS (National Forensic Laboratory
  Information System), 157
Nicotine dependence, 189
Nixon, Richard (President), **43**, 44, 45
Nonsteroidal anti-inflammatory drugs
  interactions with marijuana, **93**
Non-Transmissible Liability Index, 26
Norepinephrine reuptake inhibitors
  for treatment of marijuana addiction,
    188

Norway, 129
NREPP (National Registry of Evidence-
  based Programs and Practices), 221
Numerical Rating Scale, 83

Obama, Barack (President), 157
Ogden, David (U.S. Deputy Attorney
  General), **44**
Ogden memo, **44**
Omeprazole, 80
Ondansetron (Zofran), 83
Oregon
  indications for medical marijuana
    program enrollment and levels
    of clinical evidence, **55**
  medical marijuana program passage
    and characteristics, **49**, 204

Paclitaxel
  interactions with marijuana, **93**
Pain
  indications for medical marijuana,
    81–82
Panic disorder, 108, 109
  marijuana use and, **103**
  synthetic cannabinoids and, 159
Parents and attitude toward marijuana
  use, 26
Parkinson's disease
  indications for medical marijuana, 87
Patient
  prevention strategies for marijuana
    misuse, **202**
  reimbursement for medical mari-
    juana, 58
Peers, 26
  prevention strategies for marijuana
    misuse, **202**
Pentobarbital
  interactions with marijuana, **93**
Pharmaceutical formulations of marijuana, 73, **74–75**
Pharmacokinetics
  metabolism and, 78

of smoked and orally ingested marijuana, 78, **79**

Pharmacology. *See also* individual drug names

interventions for treatment of marijuana addiction, 185–194

Phencyclidine

psychosis and, **122**

Phenobarbital

interactions with marijuana, **93**

Physicians and liability, 59

"Plant Food," 152

Poland, 157

Policies

drug control, 40–42

history of, 42–45, **43–44**

marijuana price elasticity, 40–41

medical, 39–60

recreational, 60–64

Posttraumatic stress disorder (PTSD)

according to DSM-5, 27

indications for medical marijuana, 89–90

marijuana comorbidity and, 111

marijuana use and, 5, **103**

as qualification in medical marijuana program, 52, 66

substance use disorders and, 27

Pot. *See* Cannabinoids; Marijuana

"Potpourri," 152

Pregnancy and adverse effects of marijuana, 91–92

Preparing for the Drug Free Years program, 210

Priming effect, 107

Prize incentives contingency management, 180

Project Chill, 214, 215

Project MATCH, 181

Project STAR, 208

PROmoting School-community-university Partnerships to Enhance Resilience (PROSPER), 213, 214

Proposition 215 (California), **44**

PROSPER (PROmoting School-community-university Partnerships to Enhance Resilience), 213, 214

Protease inhibitors

interactions with marijuana, **93**

PSAs (public service announcements), 212

Psychiatric disorders

indications for medical marijuana, 87–90, 94

marijuana comorbidity and, 111–112

use of marijuana and, 5

Psychoactive drugs

regulatory categories for, 41–42

Psychosis

clinical vignette of, 119–120

co-occurrence of, 120–130

definition of, 120

differentiating primary and secondary psychotic disorders, 120–129

algorithm for determining if psychotic symptoms are caused by substance abuse, 127, **128**

DSM-5 criteria

for brief psychotic disorder, **122–123**

for schizophrenia, **124–126**

for schizophreniform disorder, **123–124**

for substance/medication-induced psychotic disorder, **126–127**

substances of abuse that can induce psychosis, 121, **122**

DSM-5 secondary causes of, 121

indications for medical marijuana, 87–88

marijuana use and, 119–148

clinical course of psychotic disorders, 140–144

impact on cessation of, 142–144

Psychosis (*continued*)
    marijuana use and (*continued*)
        clinical course of psychotic dis-
            orders (*continued*)
            impact on clinical course of,
                140–142
        pathogenesis of psychotic disor-
            ders, 130–140
            alternative explanations for
                link between marijuana
                and schizophrenia, 138–
                139
            as component cause of
                schizophrenia, 132–138,
                134–135
            directionality of marijuana-
                psychosis association,
                131–132
            increased risk of developing
                psychotic disorders, 131
            marijuana use as component
                cause of schizophrenia,
                139–140
            theories on development and
                emergence of schizo-
                phrenia, 132
        motivations for marijuana use with
            psychotic disorders, 129–130
        rates of marijuana and other sub-
            stance use disorders with psy-
            chotic disorders, 129
PTSD. *See* Posttraumatic stress disorder
Public service announcements (PSAs),
    212
Pure Food and Drug Act, **43**

Quality control of medical marijuana,
    78–79
Quinidine
    interactions with marijuana, **93**

Randomized controlled trials (RCTs)
    for cannabinoid use
        for appetite stimulation in HIV/
            AIDS patients, 81

for seizures, 84
    for symptom management in
        dementia, 86
    for treatment of marijuana addiction,
        182
Ranitidine
    interactions with marijuana, **93**
RCTs. *See* Randomized controlled trials
Reasoned action approach, 26
Recruitment effects, 22
Reefer Madness, 45, 130–131, 172
Reimbursement for medical marijuana,
    58
Relapse prevention, 178–179
Rhode Island
    indications for medical marijuana
        program enrollment and levels
        of clinical evidence, **56**
    medical marijuana program passage
        and characteristics, **50**

SAFE, for effective prevention inter-
    ventions, 203, **203**, 216, 218, 222
Safety and Innovation Act of 2012, 64–
    65
Saquinavir
    interactions with marijuana, **93**
SAMSA (Substance Abuse and Mental
    Health Services Administration),
    220
Sativex. *See* Nabiximols
Schizophrenia
    DSM-5 criteria for, **124–126**
    etiology of, 132
    marijuana use as component cause
        of, 139–140
    medical marijuana and, 87
    psychosis as component cause of,
        132–138, **134–135**
        biological gradient, **134**, 136–137
        biological plausibility, **134,** 137
        coherence, **135**, 137–138
        consistency, 133, **134**
        experiment, **135,** 137
        specificity, 133, 136

strength, **134**, 136
temporality, 133, **134**
theories on development and emergence of, 132
Schizophrenia spectrum disorder, 121–122, 144
Schizophreniform disorder
DSM-5 criteria for, **123–124**
School
prevention strategies for marijuana misuse, **202**, 206–208
"Scooby Snacks," 152
SCs. *See* Cannabinoids, synthetic
SDS (Severity of Dependence Scale), 174
Secobarbital
interactions with marijuana, **93**
Sedatives
psychosis and, **122**
Seizures
indications for medical marijuana, 83–84
Selective preventive intervention, 201
Selective serotonin reuptake inhibitors (SSRIs)
for treatment of marijuana addiction, 187
Self-medication, 27
hypothesis of psychosis and, 131, 138
Sensation Seeking Targeting (SENTAR), 212
SENTAR (Sensation Seeking Targeting), 212
Serotonin 5-HT$_3$, 83
Serotonin-norepinephrine reuptake inhibitors
for treatment of marijuana addiction, 188
Severity of Dependence Scale (SDS), 174
SFP 10–14 (Strengthening Families Program: For Parents and Youth 10–14), 210, 211
Shafer Commission Report, 45
Shared diathesis model, 139
SIPD. *See* Substance/medication-induced psychotic disorder

Sleep disturbances, 16, 171–172
indications for medical marijuana, 90
marijuana comorbidity and, 112
marijuana use and, **103**
Social anxiety disorder, 108, 109
marijuana use and, **103**
relief with marijuana, 130
Social constraints of marijuana use, 30
Spain, 143
Spasticity
indications for medical marijuana, 82–83
Speech, 121
"Spice," 165
SSRIs. *See* Selective serotonin reuptake inhibitors
Stepping stone theory, 103
Stevens, John Paul (Justice), **44**
Stimulants and psychosis, **122**
Strengthening Families Program: For Parents and Youth 10–14 (SFP 10–14), 210, 211
Substance Abuse and Mental Health Services Administration (SAMHSA), 220
Substance/medication-induced psychotic disorder (SIPD)
co-occurring drug use hypothesis, 131
description of, 121
DSM-5 criteria for, **126–127**
Substance use disorders
algorithm for determining if psychotic symptoms are caused by substance abuse, 127, **128**
bipolar disorder and, 27–28
marijuana use and risk for, 102–103, **104**
posttraumatic stress disorder and, 27
psychosis and, 121, **122**
risk factors and, 32
Suicide
marijuana risk and, 113
marijuana use and, **103**
Sweden, 157

Synesthesias, 14
Synthetic Drug Abuse Prevention Act,
    64–65, 157

Tangentiality, 121
Technology
    for self-administered substance use
        prevention programs, 215
    software-based interventions for
        treatment of marijuana addic-
        tion, 183–184
Tetrahydrocannabivarin, 73
THC. *See* Delta-9-tetrahydrocannabinol
THC-COOH, 79–80
Theophylline
    interactions with marijuana, **93**
Theory of planned behavior, 26
Thoughts, disorganized, 121
Tincture, **77**
TLI (Transmissible Liability Index),
    25–26
Tobacco and marijuana use, **103**
Topicals, **77**
Transient sensory experiences, 14
Transmissible Liability Index (TLI),
    25–26
Triazolam
    interactions with marijuana, **93**
Twin studies
    ACE models and, 23, **23**
    sequential risk model and, 105

UDS (urine drug screen), 190
Unipolar depression and marijuana
    use, **103**
United Kingdom, 157
    approved use of nabiximols, 73
    drug control policy in, 63
United Nations Single Convention on
    Narcotic Drugs, 2, **43**, 64, 65
United States. *See also* individual states
    ambivalence and controversy and,
        4–5
    marijuana use in, 4–7
Urine drug screen (UDS), 190

Uruguay, 63–64
U.S. Constitution
    Fifth Amendment, 44
U.S. Customs and Border Control, 157
U.S. Department of Justice, 6, 52
U.S. Department of Veterans Affairs
    (VA), 59–60
U.S. Drug Enforcement Administra-
    tion (DEA), 2, 58, 73, 155, 157
U.S. Food and Drug Administration
    (FDA), 4, 42, 73, 185
U.S. Supreme Court
    ruling on drug control, 44–45

VA. *See* U.S. Department of Veterans
    Affairs
Venlafaxine
    for treatment of marijuana addiction,
        188
Ventral tegmental area (VTA), 14, 17,
    18
Verapamil
    interactions with marijuana, **93**
Vermont
    indications for medical marijuana
        program enrollment and levels
        of clinical evidence, **56**
    medical marijuana program passage
        and characteristics, **50**
Vinblastine
    interactions with marijuana, **93**
Vindesine
    interactions with marijuana, **93**
Violence
    marijuana risk and, 113
    marijuana use and, **103**
Virginia
    legalization of medical marijuana,
        45–46
Vitamin B_{12}, 121
Voucher-based reinforcement, 180
VTA (ventral tegmental area), 14, 17, **18**

Warfarin
    interactions with marijuana, **93**

War on Drugs, 5, 40, **43**
Washington (D.C.)
    indications for medical marijuana
        program enrollment and levels
        of clinical evidence, **56**
    medical marijuana program passage
        and characteristics, **50**, 204
Washington (State)
    indications for medical marijuana
        program enrollment and levels
        of clinical evidence, **56**
    legalization
        of medical marijuana, 204
        of recreational marijuana, **44**
    Liquor Control Board, 62
    medical marijuana program passage
        and characteristics, **50**

sale of marijuana for recreational
        use, 62
Wild dagga (*Leonotis leonurus*), 152
Wisconsin
    legalization of medical marijuana,
        45–46
Withdrawal syndrome, 30–31
Word salad, 121

Youth and use of marijuana, 6, 8
"Yucatan Fire," 152

Zofran (Ondansetron), 83
Zolpidem
    for treatment of marijuana addiction,
        190

CPSIA information can be obtained
at www.ICGtesting.com
Printed in the USA
LVOW04s2058110316

478844LV00003B/3/P